Mental Health for Nursing

Lalit Batra M.D.
Consultant Psychiatrist and Assistant Professor (Psychiatry)
Psychiatric Centre and Department of Psychiatry
S.M.S. Medical College
Jaipur (India)

Formerly at
Institute of Human Behavior and Allied Sciences, **Delhi**
Department of Psychiatry, S.P. Medical College, **Bikaner**

PEEPEE
PUBLISHERS AND DISTRIBUTORS (P) LTD.

Mental Health for Nursing

Published by
Pawaninder P. Vij and Anupam Vij

Peepee Publishers and Distributors (P) Ltd.
Head Office: 160, Shakti Vihar, Pitam Pura, Delhi-110 034 (India)

Correspondence Address:
7/31, First Floor, Ansari Road, Daryaganj
New Delhi-110 002 (India)

Ph: 41512412, 23246245, 9811156083

e-mail: peepee160@yahoo.co.in

e-mail: peepee160@gmail.com

www.peepeepub.com

join us on facebook.com/pp.publishers

First Edition Reprint: 2020

ISBN: 81-8445-021-4
978-81-8445-021-7

To
My wife
Dr. Anju Batra,
Thanks for all times, always

Preface

This book "*Mental Health for Nursing*" is primarily aimed at nurses studying for the general as well as B.Sc. courses. It is intended to provide a broad theoretical background both for examinations and for practical work on the wards.

It is hoped that this clinical guide will help you plan realistic nursing care plans individualized to your patient's present level of functioning and priority of needs. Chapters 1 to 15 present an overview of history of psychiatric nursing, psychiatric nursing principles, psycho-social nursing care planning, clinical interview and communication skills, sign and symptoms in psychiatry and legal and ethical aspects in mental health nursing. Chapters 15 to 28 examine a full range of psychiatric syndromes and their clinical phenomena, available treatment modalities and role of nurse, various nursing assessment tools and nursing interventions and role of nurse in community mental health.

It is my mission and hope that this concise and easy to read textbook will help nursing students in understanding mental health in a better way as speciality and also help the students appearing for examinations.

I welcome comments and suggestions for improvement from readers at my e-mail address: dr_lalitbatra@hotmail.com

Lalit Batra

Acknowledgements

At the outset, I express my sincere thanks to God for giving me this opportunity and for providing strength and energy to fulfill this commitment.

During the writing of this book I sought and was freely given, the expert advice of a number of colleagues and friends. I am deeply grateful to my excellent reviewers whose background included clinicians, educators and students. Their dedication and love for this book was evident in their attention to detail and wide breadth of knowledge. Their contribution was invaluable and I thank each and every one.

Prof. Shiv Gautam, *Prof. & Head, Dept. of Psychiatry, SMS Medical College, Jaipur.*

Dr. G.N. Arora, *Retd. Principal, Govt. Autonomous College, Kota.*

Dr. Purav Middha, *MD Consultant Psychiatrist, Kothari Medical and Research Institute, Bikaner.*

Dr. Ravi Gupta, *MD Senior Resident, Dept. of Psychiatry, UCMS and GTB Hospital, Delhi.*

Dr. Amit Nijhawan, *MD Research Associate, Dept. of Psychiatry, SMS Medical College, Jaipur.*

Dr. Deepti Munshi, *MD (Student), Dept. of Psychiatry, SMS Medical College, Jaipur.*

I am grateful to my friends and colleagues Prof. (Mrs) Madhu Nijhawan, Prof. R.K. Solanki, Prof. Pradeep Sharma, Dr. (Mrs) K.Kanwal, Dr. Sanjay Jain, Dr. Paramjeet Singh, Dr. I.D. Gupta, Dr. Alok Tyagi, Dr. Anil Tambi, Dr. Suresh Gupta, Dr. D.R. Swami, Dr. Rajeev Agarwal, Dr. Yogesh Satija and Dr. Rakesh Yadav for their encouragement.

It was a pleasant experience to work with Mr. Pawaninder P. Vij, Chairman and Director of Peepee Publishers and Distributors (P) Ltd., New Delhi for this venture. *I am also thankful to* Mr. Rajat Batra of *Rajat Book Corner, Jaipur for seeing this venture to completion.*

I deeply appreciate the full cooperation of Mrs. Veena Pandey, Principal, Ms. Sushma Rani Chugh, Vice-Principal, College of Nursing, Ms. Shikha Krishnan and Ms. Smitha K.P., students, B.Sc. (Nursing), College of Nursing, Jaipur.

Finally I would like to mention my heartfelt gratitude to my parents, parents-in-law, my brothers and sons for their love and devotion. Of course above all are the sacrifice, dedication and support of my wife, Dr. Anju Batra, which helped me in taking this project to completion.

Contents

1 Mental Health and Illness

INTRODUCTION

According to World Health Organization (WHO) ***"Health" is defined as the complete physical, mental and social well-being and not merely the absence of disease or infirmity.***

A sound mind in a sound body was recognized as a social ideal for many centuries.

Mental health is often spoken of as a state of well-being associated with happiness, contentment, satisfaction, achievement, optimism or hope. These terms are difficult to define, because their meaning changes, as they relate to a particular person and life situation. Mental health cannot be confined to a simple concept or a single aspect of behavior, instead mental health incorporates a number of criteria that exist on a continuum with gradients or degrees. These criteria form the basis of the optimum of mental health. However, they are not absolute, and each person has limits. Although no one reaches the ideal in all the criteria, most people can approach the optimum.

MENTAL HEALTH

Mental health is thus the balanced development of individual's personality and emotional attitudes, which enable him to live harmoniously with his fellow men. Mental health is not exclusively a matter of the relation between persons; it is matter of relation of the individual towards the community he lives in, towards the society of which the community is a part, and towards the social institutions which, for a large part guide his life.

Thus a person who is mentally healthy, is able to deal with normal human emotions, is productive, has successful relationship with others, can adapt to change and can cope with adversity.

Criteria of Mental Health

Mental health is not merely an absence of mental illness. Mental health is the full and harmonious functioning of the whole personality. The following six criteria are the indicators of positive mental health developed by Marie Jahoda.

1. Positive attitude towards self
2. Growth, development and self actualization
3. Integration
4. Autonomy
5. Reality perception
6. Environmental mastery.

A mentally healthy person has following main characteristics:

1. He feels ***comfortable about himself,*** that is, he feels reasonably secure and adequate. He neither underestimates nor overestimates his own ability. He accepts his shortcomings. A mentally healthy person is free from internal conflicts. He is not at war with himself. He has a strong sense of self esteem.
2. He is ***well adjusted.*** He is able to get along well with others. He is able to form effective relationships. He accepts criticisms and is not easily upset. He is able to like and trust others.

3. He is ***able to meet the demands of life.*** He faces problems and tries to solve them intelligently, i.e. has the ability to cope with stress and anxiety. He is productive and sets reasonable goals for himself.

Living in a stress-free environment will pave the way for mentally healthier and happier life. In general, mental health can be achieved in many ways, like individual treatment, treatment of families and educational programmes. Sound behavior patterns can be encouraged and reinforced in a well established social network. Thus, healthy social surrounding is the need of the hour. Mental health is a positive science as it sets out to establish a condition of healthy mindedness.

NORMALITY

WHO's definition of "Health" has given normality a positive tone as against the classical definitions of normality as an antonym for illness. To identify any abnormality or deviance we must first know what is normal. This is easier said than done. The concept of normality has been a central issue of debate for decades and still unresolved. If we assume normality to be just an absence of illness, then merely absence of gross symptoms (psychopathology) may often be equated with normality.

Functional Perspectives of Normality

It is necessary to have a functional or operational definition of normality so as to identify abnormality or deviance. The behavioral or social science approach to normality describes it in four perspectives, i.e. normality as health, as utopia, as average and as interacting systems. Such perspectives are unique and each has its own definition.

1. ***Normality as Health:*** The perspective of normality as health is basically the traditional medical approach to health and illness. According to this approach a behavior is considered to be normal when no symptoms of disease are seen. Thus, it is basically a negative definition of normality. It correlates with the traditional role model of a doctor whose aim is to relieve his patient of grossly observable signs and symptoms of illness. Health in this context refers to a reasonable, rather than optimal, state of functioning.
2. ***Normality as Utopia:*** Utopia means a state of ideal perfection. Thus, this approach to normality regards it as a state of highly integrated optimal functioning. According to it, a person is said to be normal only when he has achieved his potential. This approach is highly value-laden, differs from culture to culture and seems to have no limits. It is therefore known by the terms such as utopia. Each culture has its own norms and ideals. Thus, the concept of normality as Utopia is related to the values of a particular culture.
3. ***Normality as an Average:*** This approach is based on the mathematical principle of average. According to this maximum number of persons fall in the middle. Those at the extremes are very less and hence are abnormal. Those in the middle constitute a majority and hence are normal. This approach may hold good for biological variables e.g. blood pressure, heart rate, temperature etc.

   But its utility in defining abnormal behaviors and emotions may have its pitfalls. For example, if in a school setting, a particular child, who may not be having any signs and symptoms of any illness, behaves differently from others, teacher often single him out. He may then be referred to the school counsellor. The child does not have any illness, he may even feel well, but just because his behavior is different from average, and he is seen as not normal.
4. ***Normality as an Interacting System:*** This aspect suggests that normal behavior is the result of interaction between biological (physical), psychological and social systems over time. Each of these three systems has

variables and factors which determine what is normal. The changes that take place over time in any of these systems, also play a role in determining the behavior. Thus, developmental factors are also included in this definition. Although this definition is as yet not thought of and well conceptualized, it appears to be the most comprehensive definition.

CONCLUSION

It is very important to recognize the fact that all four aspects of normality, i.e. as health, as utopia, as average and as interacting systems are not mutually exclusive, rather, all these aspects often overlap each other and are dependent on each other.

It may be concluded that "Normality" is broadly speaking a statistical term. How majority of persons in a given society behave, interact, present themselves in that given socio-cultural milieu, should be regarded as normal. Behavioral patterns away from these norms, may be regarded as deviance.

MENTAL HEALTH PROBLEMS

People without a mental illness can have mental health problems that are distressing and require treatment. Most people experience mental health problems at one or another time, especially during stressful periods, such as after a natural disaster, during wars, loss of a loved one, or during a serious illness. The term mental health problem refers to signs and symptoms of mental illnesses that don't fit in criteria for a specific disorder.

Dimension of Mental Illness

Mental disorders are prevalent all over the world irrespective of age, sex, socio-economic status and religion. There may be certain areas where particular disorders are more prevalent than others. Researchers have done number of epidemiological studies all over the world and drawn a few conclusions:

- At a given point of time 1% of population suffers from severe mental disorders like Schizophrenia and other psychosis.
- About 10% of population suffers from minor mental disorders like Anxiety, Neurotic disorders etc.
- Around 20-30% of patients in general clinical settings are suffering from an underlying psychiatric disorder.
- In India around 10-12 million persons are estimated to suffer from serious mental disorders and approximately 100 million from neurotic and psychosomatic disorders.
- Suicide rate in India is about 10 per lac population.
- Mental illnesses are a major contributor to the burden of illness in United States and nearly 50% of people aged 15-54 have had a psychiatric or substance abuse disorders in their lifetime, and close to 30% have had one of these disorders in the past one year.
- The Global Burden of Disease Study showed (in year 1996) that out of 15 leading causes of disability in developed countries, five are mental health problems: (i) Unipolar major depressive disorders (ii) Alcohol abuse (iii) Schizophrenia (iv) Self-inflicting injuries (v) Bipolar disorders.
- With regards to years lived with disability, depressive disorders as a single diagnostic category were the leading causes of disability.
- By the year 2020, mental disorders are projected to increase, and major depression is predicted to become the second leading cause of disease burden worldwide.

KEY POINTS

- According to World Health Organization (WHO) "Health" is defined as the complete physical, mental and social well-being and not merely the absence of disease or infirmity.
- Mentally healthy people are able to deal with normal human emotions.
- Mental disorders are health conditions characterized by alteration in thinking, mood or behavior and are associated with distress or impaired functioning.
- "Normality" is broadly speaking a statistical term. How majority of persons in a given society behave, interact, present themselves in that given socio-cultural milieu, should be regarded as normal.
- Normality describes it in four perspectives, i.e. Normality as Health, as Utopia, as Average and as Interacting systems.
- The term mental health problem refers to signs and symptoms of mental illnesses that do not fit in criteria for a specific disorder.
- Most people experience mental health problems at one or another, especially during stressful periods, such as after a natural disaster, during wars, loss of a loved one, or during a serious illness.
- At a given point of time 1% of population suffers from severe mental disorders like Schizophrenia and other psychosis.
- About 10% of population suffers from minor mental disorders like Anxiety, Neurotic disorders etc.
- Around 20-30% of patients in general clinical settings are suffering from an underlying psychiatric disorder.

2

Brain and Behaviors

Now it is believed that all human behavior results from action that originates in the brain and its amazing interconnection of neural networks or its ability to adopt and change in both structure and function.

This chapter reviews the basic information necessary for understanding neuroscience. It will review basic central nervous system structures and functions, basic mechanisms of neurotransmission, general function of major neurotransmitters, and neuroimaging techniques.

NEUROANATOMY AND CENTRAL NERVOUS SYSTEM

This section discusses each functioning area of the brain separately; each area is intricately connected with the others functions interactively. The total nervous system of human body includes Central Nervous System (CNS) and Peripheral Nervous System (PNS). The Central Nervous System contains the brain, brain stem and spinal cord, whereas the Peripheral Nervous System consists of neurons that connect CNS to periphery of the body (Muscles, Organ etc.). A brief review of key brain regions is presented in Figures 2.1 to 2.3.

Cerebrum

The largest part of the human brain fills the entire upper portion of cranium. The cortex or outer most surface of the cerebrum makes up about 80% the human brain. The cortex is 4 to 6 cellular layer thick and each layer is composed of cell bodies mixed with capillary blood vessels. This mixture makes the cortex grey brown and thus termed as grey matter. The cortex contains a number of bumps and grooves in fully developed brain which are called Gyri and Sulci respectively. The longest and deepest groove, the longitudinal fissure, separates the cerebrum into left and right hemispheres.

These two divisions of hemispheres are almost symmetrical.

Left and Right Hemispheres

The cerebrum can be roughly divided into two hemispheres. For most people one hemisphere is dominant, whereas about 5% of individuals have mixed dominance.

Each hemisphere controls mainly the functioning of the opposite side of the body. The left hemisphere is dominant in about 90% people and controls functions mainly on the right side of the body. The two hemispheres are connected by the corpus callosum, a bundle of neuronal tissue that allows information to be exchanged quickly between right and left hemisphere. An intact corpus callosum is required for smooth and coordinated functioning of both hemispheres.

Lobes of the Brain

The lateral surface of each hemisphere is further divided into four lobes; the frontal, parietal, temporal and occipital lobes. Each lobe of brain

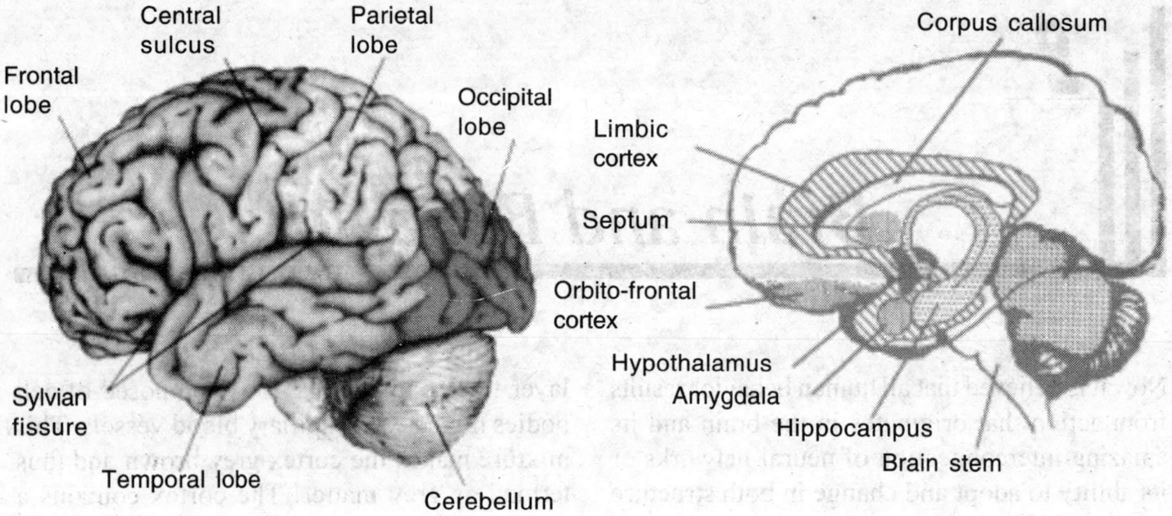

Fig. 2.1: Lateral and medial surfaces of the brain. Left, the left lateral surface of the brain. Right, the medial surface of the right half of a sagittally hemisected brain

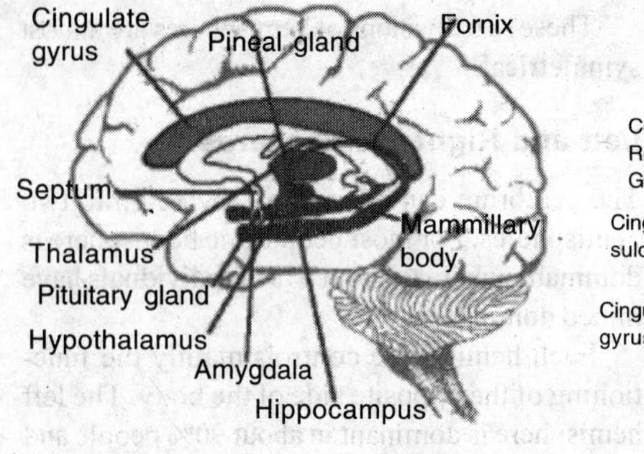

Fig. 2.2: The structures of the limbic system are integrally involved in memory and emotional behavior. (Theories link changes in the limbic system to many major mental disorders, including schizophrenia, depression, and anxiety disorders)

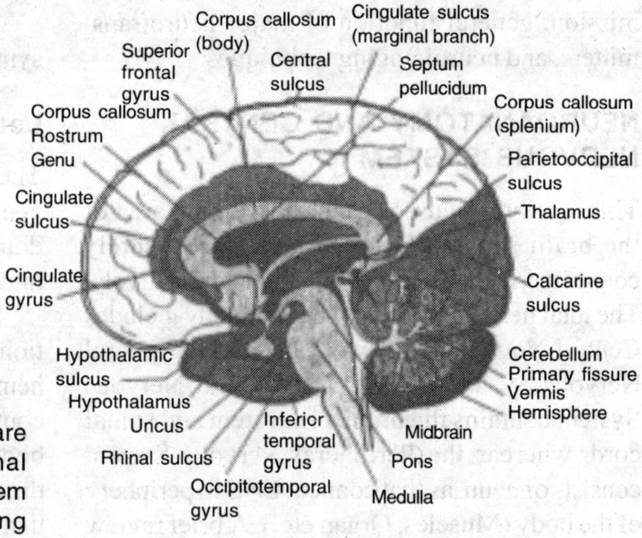

Fig. 2.3: Gyri and sulci of the cortex

is responsible for specific function, but they work in a coordinated way. Damage to specific lobes produces the symptoms of mental illness.

1. ***Frontal lobes***: The right and left frontal lobes make up about one fourth of the entire cerebral cortex and are proportionately larger in the humans than in any other mammal. The pre-central gyrus contains the ***primary motor area***. Damage to this gyrus causes spastic paralysis in the opposite side of the body. The frontal lobe also contains ***Broca's area,*** which controls the motor function of speech. Damage to Broca's area produces expressive aphasia, or difficulty with the motor movements of speech.

   Working memory is an important aspect of frontal lobe function, including the ability to plan and initiate activity with future goals in mind. Insight, judgment, reasoning, concept formation, problem solving skills, abstraction, and self evaluation are all abilities that are modulated and affected by action of the frontal lobes. These skills are often referred to as executive functions. Alterations in normal frontal lobe functioning causes deterioration in executive functioning and modulation of impulses can be lost, leading to changes in mood and personality.
2. ***Parietal lobes***: The parietal lobe contribute to the ability to recognize objects by touch, calculate, write, recognize fingers of the opposite hands, draw and organize spatial directions such as how to travel to familiar places. Damage to this area results in deficits in the ***discriminative sensory functions.*** This produces complex sensory deficits including neglect of contra lateral sensory stimuli and spatial relationships.
3. ***Temporal lobe***: The temporal lobe contains the ***primary auditory and olfactory areas***. Wernicke's area, located at the posterior aspect of the superior temporal gyrus, is primarily responsible for receptive speech.

   The temporal lobe also integrates sensory and visual information involved in control of written and verbal language skills as well as visual recognition. The hippocampus, an important structure discussed later, lies in the internal aspects of each temporal lobe and contributes to memory.
4. ***Occipital lobes***: The ***primary visual area*** is located in the most posterior aspect of the occipital lobe. Damage to this area results in a condition called cortical blindness. The occipital lobes are involved in many aspects of visual integration of information, including color vision, object and facial recognition, and the ability to perceive objects in motion.

Association Cortex

The association cortex is an important area that allows the lobes to work in an integrated manner. Areas of one lobe of the cortex often share functions with an area of the adjacent lobe.

For example, areas in the inferior parietal, posterior temporal and anterior occipital lobes integrates visual, somatosensory, and auditory information to provide the abilities required for basic academic skills. These areas, along with numerous connections beneath the cortex, are part of the mechanisms that allow the human brain to work as an integrated whole.

Sub Cortical Structures

Beneath the cortex are layers of tissues composed of the axons of cell bodies. The axonal tissue forms pathways that are surrounded by glia, a fatty or lipid substance, which have a white appearance and give these layers of axons their name—***white matter***. Structures inside the hemispheres, beneath the cortex, are considered sub cortical. Many of these structures, essential in regulation of emotions and behavior, are as follows:

1. ***Basal ganglia:*** The basal ganglia are sub cortical grey matter areas in both the right and the left hemisphere. The basal ganglia are involved with motor functions and control muscle tone, activity and posture. It co-ordinates large muscle movements and inhibit unwanted muscular activity. The basal ganglia have many connections with the cerebral cortex, thalamus, midbrain structures, and spinal cord. Damage to portions of these nuclei may produce changes in posture or muscle tone. In addition damage may produce abnormal movements, such as twitches or tremors and cause ***extra pyramidal syndromes***.
   Many of antipsychotic drugs adversely affect basal ganglia and lead to motor side effects. The ***Parkinson's disease*** is associated with a dysfunction of the basal ganglia.
2. ***Limbic System (Seat of Emotions)*****:** The limbic system is essential to understanding the many hypothesis related to psychiatric disorders and emotional behavior in general. Basic emotions, needs, drives, and instinct begin and are modulated in the limbic system. Hate, love, sex, anger, aggression and caring are basic emotions that originate within the limbic system.
   Hypothesized changes in the limbic system play a significant role in many theories of major mental disorders, including schizophrenia, anxiety and depression. The limbic system structures include the hippocampus, thalamus, hypothalamus, amygdala and limbic midbrain system. ***Kluver –Bucy syndrome*** develops when the entire limbic system is removed or destroyed.
3. ***Hippocampus:*** The hippocampus consolidates recently acquired information about facts and events, some how turning short term memory in to long term memory. It is involved in storing information, especially the emotions attached to a memory. Our emotional response to memories and our association with other related memories are function of how information is stored within the hippocampus.
   Destruction of the left hippocampus impairs verbal memory and damage to the right hippocampus results in difficulty with recognition and recall of complex visual and auditory patterns. Deterioration of the nerves of the hippocampus and other related temporal lobe structures (found in Alzheimer's disease) produces the hallmark symptoms of memory dysfunction.
4. ***Thalamus:*** Thalamus is also called the "relay-switching center of the brain." The thalamus function as a regulatory structure to relay all sensory information except smell, sent to the CNS from the PNS. From the thalamus the sensory information is relayed mostly to the cerebral cortex. The thalamus relays and regulates by filtering incoming information and determining what to pass on to the cortex. Because of its primary relay function, damage to a very small area of the thalamus may produce deficits in many cortical functions, producing behavioral abnormalities.
5. ***Hypothalamus*****:** Basic human activities such as sleep rest pattern, body temperature and physical drives such as hunger and sex, are regulated by another part of limbic system that rests deep within the brain and is called hypothalamus. It weighs only 4 grams. Dysfunction of this structure, whether from disorders or as a consequence of the adverse effect of drugs used to treat mental illness, produces common psychiatric symptoms such as appetite and sleep problems.
   Nerve cells within the hypothalamus secret the hormones-antidiuretic and oxytocin. The pituitary gland, often called the master gland, is directly connected by thousands of neurons that attach it to the ventral aspect of the hypothalamus. Together with the pituitary gland the hypothalamus functions as one of

the primary regulators of many aspects of the endocrine system. Its functions are involved in controlling of visceral activities, such as body temperature, arterial blood pressure, hunger, thirst, fluid balance, gastric motility and gastric secretions.

6. ***Amygdala***: The amygdala is directly connected with more primitive centers of the brain involving the sense of smell. It has numerous connections to the hypothalamus and lies adjacent to the hippocampus. The amygdala provides emotional component to memory and is involved in modulating aggression and sexuality. Impulsive acts of aggression and violence have been linked to dysregulation of the amygdala.
7. ***Limbic Midbrain Nuclei***: The limbic midbrain nuclei are a collection of neurons that appear to play a role in the biologic basis of addiction, sometimes referred to as the pleasure center or reward center of the brain. Emotions such as feeling satisfied with good food, the pleasure of nurturing young and the enjoyment of sexual activity originate in limbic midbrain nuclei. When functioning in abnormal ways, the limbic midbrain nuclei can begin to reinforce unhealthy or risky behaviors, such as drug abuse.

Other Central Nervous System Structures

The ***extra pyramidal motor system*** is a bundle of nerve fibers connecting the thalamus to basal ganglia and cerebral cortex. Muscle tone, common reflexes, and automatic voluntary motor functioning, such as walking are controlled by this nerve track. Dysfunction of this motor track can produce hyper tonicity in muscle groups. In Parkinson's disease, the cells that compose extra pyramidal motor system are severely affected, producing many involuntary motor movements

The ***pineal body*** is located above and medial to the thalamus. Because the pineal gland easily calcifies, it can be visualized by neuroimaging and often is a medial landmark. Its function remains somewhat a mystery. It contains secretary cells that emit the neurohormone melatonin and other substances. These hormones are thought to have a number of regulatory functions within the endocrine system. Information received from light-dark sources control release of melatonin, which has been associated with sleep and emotional disorders.

The ***locus ceruleus*** is a tiny cluster of neurons that fan out and innervate almost every part of the brain including most of the cortex, the thalamus and hypothalamus, cerebellum and the spinal cord. Just one neuron from the ceruleus can connect to more than 250,000 other neurons.

Because of its wide ranging connections, this tiny structure has the influence in the regulation of attention, time perception, sleep rest cycle, arousal, learning, pain and mood and is most involved with information processing of new unexpected and novel experience. Some think that its function/dysfunction may explain why individuals become addicted to substance and seek out risky behaviors, despite awareness of negative consequences.

The **brain stem** located beneath the thalamus and composed of midbrain, pons and medulla, has important life sustaining functions. Nuclei of numerous neural pathway to the cerebrum are located in the brain stem. They are significantly involved in mediating symptoms of emotional dysfunction. These nuclei are also the primary source of several neurochemicals, such as serotonin that are commonly associated with psychiatric disorders.

The ***cerebellum*** is located in the posterior aspect of the skull, beneath the cerebral hemisphere. This large structure controls movement and postural adjustments. To regulate postural balance and positioning the cerebellum receives information from all part of the body, including joints, skin and visceral organs as well as from many parts of the CNS.

Autonomic Nervous System (ANS) is closely associated with the spinal cord, but not lying entirely within its columns. It is a subdivision of PNS.

This system contains efferent nerves, or motor system neurons, which affect target tissues such as cardiac muscle, smooth muscle and the glands. It also contains afferent nerves, which are sensory and conduct information from these organs back to the CNS. The autonomic nervous system is further divided into the sympathetic and parasympathetic nervous systems (See Fig. 2.4).

NEUROTRANSMITTERS

Neurotransmitters are key factors in understanding how various regions of the brain function and how interventions, such as medications and other therapies, affect brain activity and human behavior.

Neurotransmitters are manufactured in the neuron and released from the axon, or presynaptic cell, which is the space between neurons. This neurotransmission process makes communication between brain cells possible. Like a key inserted into a lock, each of these chemicals fits precisely into specific receptor cells embedded in the membrances of the axons and dendrites.

Depending on the chemical makeup of the neurotransmitters, the signal it gives either excites the receiving cells, causing them to produce an action, or inhibits the receiving cells, which slows or stops an action. After release into the synapse and communication with receptor cells, the neurotransmitters are transported back from the synapse into the axon in a process called reuptake, where they are stored for future use or are inactivated (metabolized) by enzymes.

The nervous system cells are surrounded by myelin sheaths formed by specialized groups of cells called glial cells. These are support cells that insulate neurons, remove excess transmitters and ions from the extra cellular spaces in the brain, provide glucose to some nerve cells, and direct the flow of blood and oxygen to various parts of brain.

Several chambers (ventricles) within the brain carry fluid (cerebro-spinal fluid). The cerebral spinal fluid (CSF) cushions, protects and bathes the brain and spinal cord, carrying chemicals, nutrients, and waste to and fro the blood stream.

From this basic explanation it is evident that neurons are very specialized, and neurotransmitters perform vital functions in the normal working brain. Their absence or excess can play a major role in the brain disease and behavioral disorders. A single neurotransmitters can effect other brain chemicals as well as several different subtypes of receptor cells, each located along tracks connecting different regions of the brain. Thus the same neurotransmitter can have one effect in one part of the brain and different effects in another part of the brain.

Nearly all of the known neurotransmitters fall into one of the two categories: small amine molecules (monoamines, acetyl-choline, and amino acids) and peptides. Few important neurotransmitters are described in Table 2.1.

NEUROIMAGING TECHNIQUES

Until the last few decades the only way to directly study the brain was through surgery, open head trauma, or autopsy. Brain imaging techniques allow direct viewing of the structure and function of the intact, living brain. These techniques help not only in diagnosing some brain disorders but also in mapping the region of the brain, measuring the activity or function in these regions, and correlating this activity with the effect of

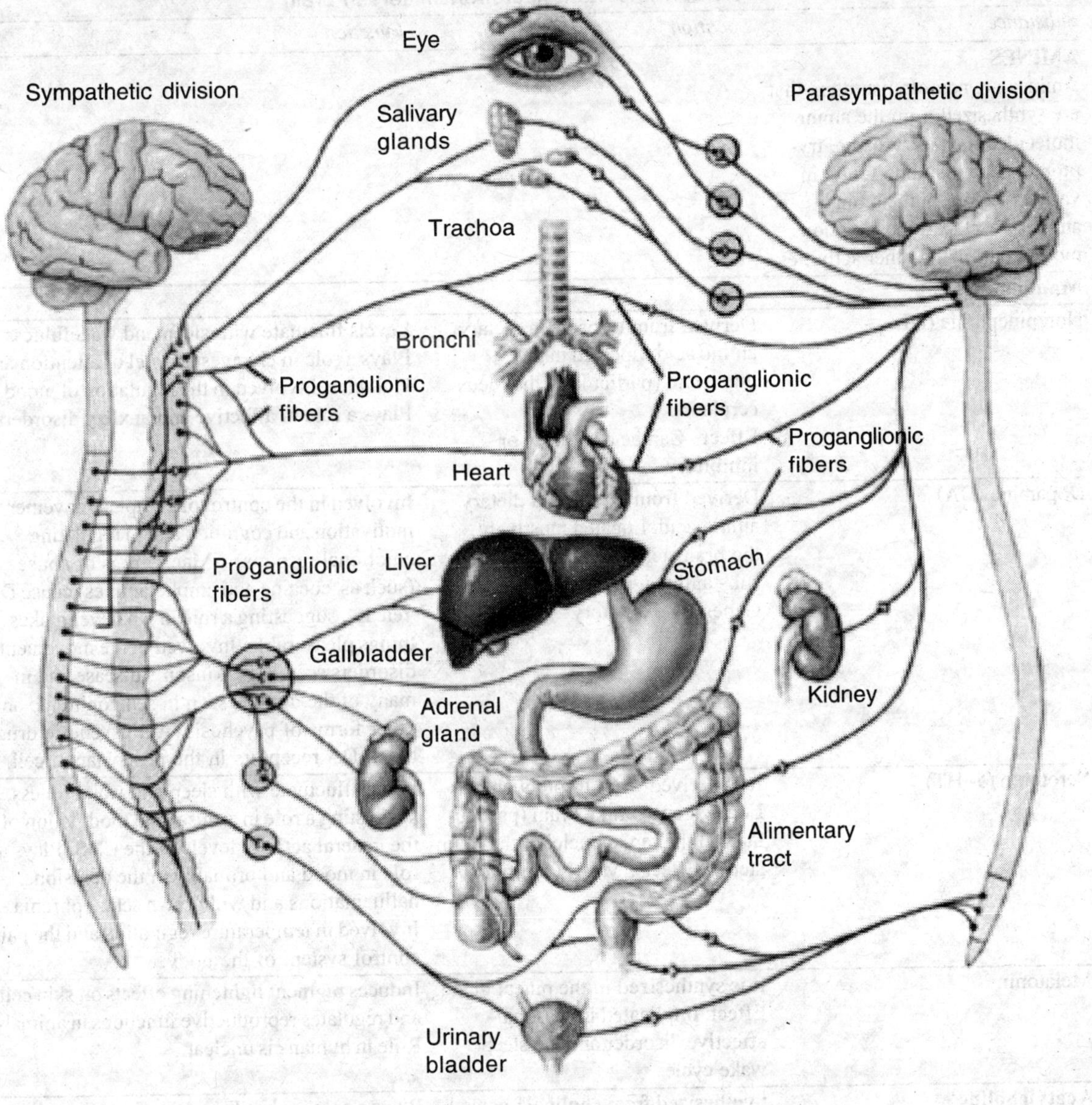

Fig. 2.4: Diagram of the autonomic nervous system

interventions. Two basic neuroimaging methods are structural and functional neuroimaging.

Structural Neuroimaging

Commonly used structure neuroimaging techniques include ***computed tomography*** (CT) and ***magnetic resonance imaging*** (MRI), which permit visualization of brain structures. They can detect structural abnormalities, changes in the volume of brain tissue, and enlargement of the cerebral ventricles. They do not reveal anything about how the brain works.

Table 2.1: Important neurotransmitters in brain

Substance	*Location*	*Function*
AMINES Amines are neurotransmitters that are synthesized from the amino molecules such as tyrosine, tryptophan and histidine found in various regions of the brain, amines affect learning, emotions motor control and other activities.		
Monoamines		
Norepinephrine (NE)	Derived from tyrosine, a dietary amino acid. Located in the brainstem (particularly the locus ceruleus). Effect : Can be excitatory or inhibitory.	Levels fluctuate with sleep and wakefulness. Plays a role in changes in level of attention and vigilance. Involved in the regulation of mood. Plays a role in affective and anxiety disorders.
Dopamine (DA)	Derived from tyrosine, a dietary amino acid. Located mostly in the brainstem (particularly the substantia nigra). Effect: Generally excitatory	Involved in the control of complex movements, motivation and cognition and in regulating emotional responses. Many drugs of abuse (such as cocaine and amphetamines) cause DA release, suggesting a role in whatever makes things pleasurable. Involved in the movement disorders seen in Parkinson's disease and in many of the deficits seen in schizophrenia and other forms of psychosis. Antipsychotic drugs block DA receptors in the postsynaptic cell.
Serotonin (5- HT)	It is derived from tryptophan. Located only in the brain (particularly in the raphe nuclei of the brainstem). Effect : Mostly inhibitory.	Levels fluctuate with sleep and wakefulness, suggesting a role in arousal and modulation of the general activity levels of the CNS. Plays a role in mood and probably in the delusions, hallucinations and withdrawn schizophrenia. Involved in temperature regulation and the pain control system of the body.
Melatonin	It is synthesized in the pineal gland. Effect: Implicated in seasonal affective disorder and the sleep wake cycle.	Induces pigment lightening effects on skin cells and regulates reproductive functions in animals. Role in humans is unclear.
Acetylcholine	Synthesized from choline. Located in the brain and spinal cord but is more widespread in the peripheral nervous system, particularly the neuromuscular junction of skeletal muscle. Effect: Can have an excitatory or inhibitory effect	Plays a role in the sleep-wakefulness cycle. Alzheimer's disease is associated with the decrease in aetylcholine-secretin neurons. Myasthenis gravis (weakness of skeletal muscles) results from a reduction in acetylcholine receptors.
Amino acids Gamma-aminobutyric acid (GABA)	A glutamate derivative; most neurons of the CNS have receptors. Effect: Major transmitter for postsynaptic inhibition on the CNS.	Drugs that increase GABA function, such as the benzodiazepines, are used to treat anxiety and to induce sleep.

Functional Neuroimaging

Brain function can be studied using other imaging techniques to determine both normal activity and malfunctioning in specific regions. Techniques that study brain function includes ***brain electrical activity mapping*** (BEAM), which measures sensory inputs; and ***single photon emission computed tomography*** (SPECT), which permits the study of brain metabolism and cerebral blood flow.

Positron emission tomography (PET), SPECT and the newer functional magnetic resonance imaging (fMRI) techniques can measure the use of glucose (glucose utilization) and the amount of blood flowing in a region of brain. The more blood will flow through it, the more glucose it will use, and the brighter (yellow, orange, red) the imaging scans look.

When these techniques are coupled with neuropsychological test results, deficit in a person's performance, such as language or cognitive and sensory information processing, can be linked to the activity of the region of the brain responsible for those functions.

KEY POINTS

- The total nervous system of human body includes **Central Nervous System** (CNS) and **Peripheral Nervous System.**
- The Central Nervous System contains the brain, brain stern and spinal cord, whereas the Peripheral Nervous System consists of neurons that connect CNS to periphery of the body (Muscles, Organ etc.).
- **Executive functions** such as Insight, judgment, reasoning, concept formation, problem solving skills, abstraction, and self evaluation are all abilities that are modulated and affected by action of the **frontal lobes.**
- The **parietal lobe** contribute to the ability to recognize objects by touch, calculate, write, recognize fingers of the opposite hands, draw and organize spatial directions such as how to travel to familiar places.
- Temporal lobe contains the **primary auditory and olfactory areas**.
- The **primary visual area** is located in the most posterior aspect of the occipital lobe.
- The **basal ganglia** are involved with motor functions and control muscle tone, activity and posture. It co-ordinate large muscle movements and inhibit unwanted muscular activity.
- Basic emotions, needs, drives, and instinct begin and are modulated in the limbic system.
- **Limbic System** structures include the hippocampus, thalamus, hypothalamus, amygdala and limbic midbrain.
- The **Hippocampus** consolidates recently acquired information about facts and events, some how turning short term memory in to long term memory.
- **The Thalamus** functions as a regulatory structure to relay all sensory information except smell, sent to the CNS from the PNS.
- Basic human activities such as sleep rest pattern, body temperature and physical drives such as hunger and sex, are regulated by another part of limbic system that rests deep within the brain and is called **hypothalamus.**

- **Limbic Midbrain Nuclei** play a role in the biological basis of addiction, sometimes referred to as the pleasure center or reward center of the brain.
- Neurotransmitters are key factors in understanding how various regions of the brain function and how interventions, such as medications and other therapies, affect brain activity and human behavior.
- **Computed tomography** (CT) and **magnetic resonance imaging** (MRI), permit visualization of brain structures.
- Brain function can be studied by using imaging techniques **brain electrical activity mapping** (BEAM), **Positron emission tomography** (PET), and **single photon emission computed tomography** (SPECT).

3 Theoretical Concepts of Personality Developments and Psychiatric Nursing

PERSONALITY

Personality is a complex pattern of characteristics, largely outside of person's awareness, that comprise the individual's distinctive pattern of perceiving, feeling, thinking, coping and behaving. The personality emerges from a complicated interaction of biological dispositions, psychological experiences and environmental situations.

Normal personality is identified as what is statistically common and what is not abnormal. From the structural point of view, personality has got three components:

I. Temperament	:	Biological component
II. Character	:	Social and environmental component
III. Intelligence	:	Correlates and controls overall expression of both components.

From the moment of conception, our development is influenced by forces that ultimately shape the way in which we respond to the world around us. A person's natural tendencies are the result of a combined genetic transmission of personality traits from both parents. A unique blend of multi generational family partners is inherited though this genetic factor. There are also many societal and environmental factors that influence personality. Patterns of behavior are formed as one responds to the awareness and perception of the self as autonomous and capable of individual control.

THEORIES OF PERSONALITY DEVELOPMENT AND NURSING CARE

Why do we think and behave in a way you do?

This issue wondered many and led to integral concept in the study of psychology. These theories are the foundation of therapeutic approaches to the management of mental disorders. Nursing practice is also based on these theoretical concepts. These theories of personality development guide us in understanding of human behavior and help us in the implementing the nursing care plan effectively on patients. This chapter presents an overview of some theoretical concepts used by mental health professionals.

Psychoanalytic Theory

Concepts derived from psychoanalysis are applied so widely in psychiatric training and practice that they have become a fundamental part of the approach to mental and emotional disorders. Sigmund Freud established the basis for psychodynamic thinking. Traditionally psychoanalysis is referred primarily to be based on Freud's libido and instinct theories. Essentially the psychoanalysis is based on the free association method of investigation, through which gathered information is used to formulate the key concepts of unconscious motivations.

Sigmund Freud

Sigmund Freud was born of Jewish parents on May 6, 1856, in Freiburg, a small town in Moravia.

When he was 4 years old, his father, a wool merchant, brought the family to Vienna where Freud lived most of his life. He was forced to flee to England in 1938, when the Nazis annexed Austria. Freud died in 1939.

From 1887 to 1897, the period in which Freud seriously began to study the disturbances of his hysterical patients, psychoanalysis can be said to have taken root. The emergence of psychoanalysis had a three fold aspect: (a) A method of investigation (b) as a therapeutic technique (c) as a body of scientific knowledge based on an increasing fund of information and basic theoretical propositions.

Free Association

The method of free association, involves a patient who is instructed to say everything that comes to his/her mind, regardless of contents of importance. This in turn provides the therapist with themes arising from unconscious wishes and fears. Similar themes can be found in the recall of dreams and early childhood memories.

Theories of Freud

1. **Theory of instincts:**
   Freud used the term libido to refer to that force by which the sexual instinct is represented in the mind. Freud believed that during the first five years of life the individual progresses through several developmental periods called psychosexual stages.
   Oral stage: The first stage of life constitutes the oral stage of psychosexual development. During this period, infants derive pleasure from nursing and sucking.
   Anal stage: The second stage of life, the anal stage, is the period where children have their first experience of imposed control in the form of toilet training.
   Phallic stage: In the third stage called the phallic stage (age 3 to 6 years), children begin to derive pleasure from fondling their genitals. The penis becomes the organ of principal interest to children of both sexes. Freud believed that in phallic stage, children experienced sexual impulses toward the parent of opposite sex. This, in the case of a boy will be directed toward the mother. This leads him to perceive his father as a rival for his mother's affection. Freud termed this the "**Oedipal Conflict**." The boy then fears that his father will retaliate against these sexual impulses by castrating him, which is called the castration anxiety. Freud believed that this is the basis of all later anxieties provoked by forbidden internal desires. In normal development, the boy overcomes this by identifying with his father and internalizing an idealized perception of his father's attitude and values. This successful resolution of the oedipal conflict coincides with, and leads to, the acquisition of conscience and moral ideas (the superego).
   Latency period: The fourth stage, the latency period, lasts from about age 7 to age 12, when children gain the skills needed for coping with the environment.
   Genital stage: Adolescence and puberty marks the genital stage, when the mature phase of adult sexual concerns and pleasures are experienced.
   Freud argued that problems at any stage could arrest further development and the individual gets fixated at that stage resulting in a lasting effect on the individual's personality. Thus a person fixated in the oral stage is called an oral personality and may be fond of oral pleasures such as eating or smoking. A person fixated at the anal stage is characterized by concern with cleanliness, orderliness, saving

etc., and is called the anal personality. Failure to resolve the oedipal conflict can lead to a weak sense of morality, and difficulties with authority figures.

2. **Topographic theory:**
   The topographic theory represented an attempt to divide the mind into three regions: the unconscious, the preconscious, the conscious, which were differentiated by their relationship to consciousness.

   The unconsciousness: The Unconsciousness contains repressed ideas and affects
   1. Ordinarily the elements of unconscious are inaccessible to consciousness; they become conscious only through the preconscious, which excludes them by means of censorship or repression. Repressed ideas may reach consciousness when the censor is overpowered (as in psychoneurotic symptom formation), relaxed (as in dream state), or fooled (as in jokes).
   2. The unconsciousness is associated with a particular form of mental activity that Freud called the primary process or pleasure principle.

   The preconscious: This region of mind is not present at birth but develops in childhood. The preconscious is accessible to both the unconscious and conscious. One of the functions of preconscious is to repress or censor a person's wishes or desire. This type of mental activity is called secondary process. The secondary process thinking is closely allied with reality principle.

   The conscious: Freud regards the conscious as an organ of attention, operating in close association with the preconscious. Through attention, the person becomes conscious of perceptual stimuli from the outside world.

3. **Structural theory:**
   Freud divided the personality into three major components:
   - The id
   - The ego
   - The superego

   The id
   This is the most primitive part and is present in the newborn infant. It consists of the basic biological impulses or drives such as the need to eat, drink, eliminate waste, avoid pain, gain sexual (sensual) pleasure, aggression etc. The id seeks immediate gratification of these impulses and operates on the pleasure principle (obtain pleasure and avoid pain, regardless of the external circumstances).

   The ego
   The ego develops as the young child learns to consider the demands of reality, and learn that their impulses cannot always be gratified immediately.
   It follows the reality principle, i.e., the gratification of impulses must be delayed until the appropriate environmental conditions are met. The ego acts as the mediator between the wishes of the id and the demands of the superego.

   The superego
   The superego, is the internalized representation of the values and morals of the parents, the society etc. it is essentially the individual's conscience. The superego (conscience) determines whether an action is right or wrong, and strives for perfection. Violating the superego's standards, or even the impulse to do so, produces anxiety. This anxiety is unconscious and may be felt as guilt.

4. **Defense mechanisms:**
   Defense mechanisms are mental processes which are generally unconscious and which serve the purpose of protecting the individual from anxiety generated by intrapsychic conflicts. They are also known as **Coping Mechanism.** They are described in detail in Chapter 4.

Other Psychoanalytical Theorists

Much of Freud's theory is still used by psychotherapists. The theorists who followed him have modified and built on the original psychoanalytical theories. The index given below lists several other psychoanalytical theorists and gives a brief statement identifying the major contributions of each.

Contemporary psychoanalytical theorists

Erik Erikson (1963): Expanded Freud's theory of psychosocial development to encompass the entire life cycle.

Anna Freud (1966): Expanded psychoanalytical theory in the area of child psychology.

Melanie Klein (1949): Extended the use of psychoanalytical techniques to work with young children through development to play therapy.

Karen Horney (1950): Focused on psychoanalytical theory in terms of cultural and interpersonal factors; rejected Freud's view of feminine sexuality.

Alfred Adler: First defected from Freud and founded school of individual psychology, believed that the motivating force in human life is a sense of inferiority.

PSYCHOSOCIAL DEVELOPMENTAL THEORY

Eric Erikson

Here, instead of psychosexual functions, Erikson gives emphasis to psychosocial stages of development involving ego processes. For example, the important feature of the first year of life is not that it focuses on oral gratification, but that the child is learning to trust (versus mistrust) the environment, based on the type of the nurturing the child receives during this period. Similarly, in the second year of life, instead of focusing on anal concerns such as toilet training, the child is learning autonomy (versus shame). Erikson's theory covers the entire life span, as follows:

Erikson's psychosocial stages of development

Stage	*Psychosocial processes*	*Successful outcome*
1. Oral sensory (0-1year)	Trust vs Mistrust	Basic Trust
2. Muscular oral (1-3 years)	Autonomy vs Shame	Control over
3. Locomotor genital (3-5 yrs)	Initiative vs Guilt	Goal and purpose
4. Latency (5-11 years)	Industry vs Inferiority	Competence
5. Adolescence (11-18 years)	Identity vs Role confusion	Identity, fidelity
6. Young adulthood (18-35 years)	Intimacy vs Isolation	Commitment, love
7. Adulthood (35-50 years)	Generatively vs Stagnation	Productivity
8. Maturity (above 50 years)	Ego integrity vs Despair	Wisdom

COGNITIVE DEVELOPMENTAL THEORIES

Jean Piaget

The noted Swiss psychologist Jean Piaget (1896-1980) formulated a comprehensive theory of cognitive or intellectual development in which he described how children think and acquire knowledge. He referred to his theory of development as genetic epistemology because it studied the acquisition, modification and growth of abstract ideas and abilities; based on an inherited or biological substrate. There is a replacing of physical acts and experiences by mental ones.

Central to Piaget's theory is the concept of epigenesis, which holds that growth and development occur in a series of stages, each of which is built upon the successful mastery of the one that comes before. Every stage occurs at a certain age, and the child demonstrates a higher level of thinking during each successive stage of development.

The Process of Adaptation

Adaptation is the ability of the person to adjust to the environment through two complementary processes: assimilation and accommodation. Assimilation is a subjective process that involves the filtering of the world through one's own system of knowledge. Accommodation involves the adjustment of one's knowledge to the reality demands of the environment by recognizing or modifying the existing cognitive structure. Taken together, they enable the infant or child to adapt to the outside world and react with increasingly complex patterns of awareness and behavior called organization.

Organization is both biological and psychological, and all species inherit the ability to organize.

Stages in the Development of Intelligence

Piaget described four major stages leading to the capacity for adult thought. Each stage is a necessary prerequisite for the one that follows. The four stages are: (i) Sensorimotor stage, (ii) Stage of preoperational thought, (iii) Stage of concrete operations, and (iv) Stage of formal operations.

Sensorimotor Stage (Birth to 2 years)

Piaget used the term "sensorimotor" to describe this stage because the infant first begins to learn through sensory observation and gains control of his motor functions through activity, exploration, and manipulation of the environment.

Stage of Preoperational Thought (2 to 7 years)

During this stage, the child used symbols and language more extensively than in the sensorimotor stage. Thinking and reasoning is on an intuitive level in that the child learns without the use of reasoning. The child is unable to think logically or deductively and concepts are primitive; he can name objects, but not classes. Preoperational thought is a midway between socialized adult thought and the completely autistic Freudian unconscious.

Stage of Concrete Operations

This stage is so named because in this period the child operates and acts upon the concrete, real and perceivable world of objects and events. Egocentric thought is replaced by operational thought, which involves attending to and dealing with a wide array of information outside the child. Therefore, a child can now see a thing from someone else's perspective. Children in this stage begin to use limited logical thought processes and are able to serialize order and group things in classes based on common characteristics.

Interpersonal Theory

The theorist who originated the interpersonal model is **Harry Stack Sullivan**, a twentieth century American therapist (1953,1954). Since then it has been further developed and refined by **Gerald Klerman (1993)**, attention is also given to the interpersonal nursing theory of **Hildegard Peplau (1952)**. Her work on the psychotherapeutic role of the nurse in the interrelationship is a milestone in the field.

The goal of interpersonal therapy is to reduce symptoms, improve social functioning, and assist the person in developing more adaptive ways of relating to others. It is particularly effective with issues related to grief, role disputes, role transition and interpersonal deficits.

Harry S. Sullivan (1892-1949)

Nurses in the mental health setting develop therapeutic relationships with patients in an attempt to help them develop the ability to interact successfully with others. Sullivan believed that behavior and personality developments are the direct results of these interpersonal relationships.

Sullivan believed that human behavior could be seen in the social interaction between people.

Sullivan divided development into six stages. During infancy (birth to 18 months), the child is concerned with oral satisfaction of needs; in childhood (18 months to 6 years), children learn to delay personal gratification with a minimum of anxiety. The juvenile (6 to 9 years) is learning to develop satisfaction in relationships with the peer group while the preadolescent (9 to 12 years) is striving to develop successful interactions with persons of the same sex. During early adolescence (12 to 14 years) a sense of personal identity is formed as relationship with persons of the opposite sex are sought. In late adolescence (14 to 21 years) the person is working to develop satisfying and meaningful long term relationships with others.

Sullivan believed that the attainment of successful interpersonal relationship was dependent on the formation of interaction skills at each level of development.

Sullivan's stages of development

Stage	*Signs of successful resolution*	*Indicators of development problem*
Sullivan (Interpersonal)		
1. Infant	Satisfaction of need	Anxiety develops as a result of unmet physiologic needs
2. Childhood	Self-control in gratification	Increasing anxiety needs experienced with delay in gratification of own needs
3. Juvenile	Successful relationships with peer group	Difficulty with relating to others and developing interpersonal group relationships/workplace interaction
4. Preadolescence	Appropriate interactions with persons of opposite sex	Inability to relate in a meaningful way to persons of opposite sex
5. Early adolescence	Sense of personal identity in heterosexual relationship	Fear and withdrawal of relationships with persons of opposite sex.
6. Late adolescence	Satisfying intimate relationship with another	Inability to form a longterm intimate relationship with another person

HILDEGARD PEPLAU (1909-1999)

Hildegard Peplau, USA, provided the much needed scholarly leadership for psychiatric nurses and applied the interpersonal theory to nursing and the nurse-patient relationship. She saw the stages of developmental growth of Sullivan's theory as the basis for therapeutic interaction with patients, including many whose behaviors reflect failure to understand their own feelings and actions.

Peplau's theory identified four stages of development. In infancy, the child is learning to count on others, while the toddler is learning to delay self-gratification. At the same time, the toddler derives much pleasure in a positive response from others to his or her action. Early childhood is a time of developing the skill of behaving in a way that is acceptable to others, preceding late childhood in which the child learns to compromise, compete and co-operate in participation and interaction with others.

BEHAVIOR THEORY

B.F. Skinner (1904-1990)

One of the most influential behaviorists B.F. Skinner recognized two different kinds of learning, each evolved separate kind of behavior. According to this all behavior is observable and learned behavior in response to a stimulus from the environment. Behavior is the result of conditioning shaped by system of reward, punishment and reinforcement. Human personality is formed in response to these stimulus-response situations. The personality may include both adaptive and maladaptive behavior as the result of reinforcement. Person shows consistent patterns of behavior that will continue if the action is rewarded by a response. If no reinforcement is given, the behavior will decline.

For example, if a child climbs on a chair, reaches the faucet, and is able to get a drink of water successfully, it is more likely that the child will repeat the behavior.

COGNITIVE THEORY

Albert Bandura

Acquiring behaviors by learning from other people is the basis of social cognitive theory developed by Albert Bandura. Bandura developed his ideas after being concerned about violence on television contributing to aggression in children. He believed that personality is largely shaped through learning by actively seeking out and the process information about the environment in response to a need for a positive outcome. Social learning is based on observation and imitation of others. Both children and adults tend to imitate people they like or respect more than those whose persona is less appealing. Models whose behavior leads to an approved outcome are also more likely to be copied. An important concept of Bandura is self-efficacy, a person's sense of his or her ability to deal effectively with the environment. Efficacy beliefs influence how people feel, think, motivate themselves and behave. The stronger the self-efficacy, the higher the goals set for themselves and firmer their commitment to them.

Aron Beck

American psychiatrist Aron T. Beck devoted his career to understanding the relationship between the cognition and mental health. He focuses on the person's ability to think, analyze, and decide on certain behavior rather than acting on feeling. He realized the importance of cognition when treating people with depression, finding that the depression improved when patients began to think differently. He believed that people with depression had faulty information-processing system that leads to biased cognitions. These faulty beliefs cause error in judgment that become habitual error in thinking. These individuals incorrectly interpret life situations, and jump to inaccurate conclusions. Beck and his colleagues developed cognitive therapy, a successful approach for treatment of depression. According to Beck, negative self-talk can be changed into more positive thoughts, leading to a more positive self image and more productive outcomes.

HUMANISTIC THEORY

Humanistics view the developing person as a whole, a totality of the physical, emotional, spiritual, intellectual, and social aspects of life, that influence us towards reaching our potential. This holistic view of human being is the foundation of the nursing model of comprehensive health care delivery.

ABRAHAM MSLOW

A humanistic psychologist, theorized that one act in response to perceived internal or external force determined by certain needs that are unchanging and innate in origin. He defined these needs as a hierarchy in which some needs are more basic or more powerful than others, and as these needs are satisfied, we can move upward to meet other higher needs. It was his opinion that we cannot move to a higher level need unless the previous level of needs is satisfied. He believed that we have the unique ability to make conscious choices to seek certain things that provide value or meaning, which results in a personal identity.

WILLIAM GLASSER

The founder of Reality therapy and control theory, described four basic psychologic needs that determine our behavioral response in any given situation. He identified these as the need for love and belonging, power and fun, which we must satisfy continually. The need to love and belonging is internal, a hunger or void that may be filled by other people, pets, or even inanimate objects. Our drive of power often conflicts which our need for love as we seek to exert control over our world.

Dr. Glasser advocates that we have a choice regarding how to behave. From the moment of birth, we accumulate mental pictures from our experience with the environment. This photo album provides the basic for our choices to behave in response to a given situation. Glasser asserted that we deny the reality of a situation instead of meeting needs in a way that is responsible and within the boundaries of social norms and morality. He found that mental health is improved when we learn to meet our needs with responsible choices.

KEY POINTS

- Theories of personality development guide us in the understanding of human behaviour. Nursing practice is also based on these theoretical concepts.
- Traditionally psychoanalysis is primarily based on Ferud's libido and instinct theories.
- Free association involves a patient who is instructed to say everything that comes to his/her mind, regardless to contents of importance.
- Freud's work includes theory of instrincts (Psychosexual development), topographic theory of mind (unconscious, preconscious and conscious), structural theory of mind (Id, Ego and Supergo) and interpretation of dreams.
- Ego is psychic apparatus that is the mediator between the id and supergo, it is determined by reality principal.
- Sigmund Freud coined the idea of defense functions in 1894, but the first systematic study of defense used by ego was presented in Anna Freud's book "The Ego and the Mechanism of Defense."
- Eric Erikson gave theory of Psychosocial development, which include eight stages.
- Jean Piaget formulated a comprehensive theory of cognitive or intellectual development in which he described how children think and acquire knowledge. This theory is also referred as genetic epistemology.
- Harry S. Sullian believed that behaviour and personality developments are the direct results of interpersonal relationships. Sullivan divided development of successful interpersonal relationship into six stages.
- Hildegard Peplau provided scholarly leadership for psychiatric nurses and applied the interpersonal theory to nursing and nurse-patient relationship.
- According to Skinner that all behaviour are learned behaviour in response to a stimuli from the environment. Behaviour is the result of conditioning shaped by system of rewards, punishment and reinforcement.
- Aron T. Beck described understanding the relationship between the cognition and mental health.

4 Defense Mechanisms

Defense mechanisms are mental processes which are generally unconscious and which serve the purpose of protecting the individual from anxiety generated by intrapsychic conflicts. They are also known as **Coping Mechanism.** Sigmund Freud first identified a unique set of coping strategies that he called Ego Defense Mechanisms. Important characteristics of Defense Mechanisms are as follows:

- Defense Mechanisms or mental processes are at unconscious level and are not used deliberately.
- They protect the person from anxiety and /or resolve conflicts by modifying or changing one's behavior.
- They protect the person from negative emotions by boosting self esteem or self enhancement.

All of us at times use defense mechanisms. Use of Defense Mechanisms is a normal process of adjustment. However, sometime use of these mechanisms can also interfere with proper decision making which may give rise to psychiatric disorders.

Psychotic or the mentally ill patients having disorders of affect, thought, and perception commonly use various defense mechanism like projection, denial, distortion, regression and turning against self. Neurotic patients use commonly the defense mechanisms of conversion, displacement, dissociation, isolation, reaction formation and repression etc.

The following are examples of various commonly used defense mechanisms.

NARCISSISTIC DEFENSES (Defenses which are used by children and psychotics)

Denial: The existence of something that can induce a conflict is denied. For example, we often read about accidents/deaths etc. but we use the defense of denial to prevent the painful awareness of reality that these things cannot occur to ourselves.

The use of denial as a defense can be noticed in persons with alcoholism, who often state the consumption of alcohol has never been a problem with them. Similarly, the initial reaction to the diagnosis of a threatening illness like cancer is the example of denial.

Projection: In this defense, the person attributes his unacceptable feelings/desires/deficiencies to the external world. A well-known proverb exemplifies this "A bad workman quarrels with his tools".

Distortion: Grossly reshaping external reality to suit inner needs, including unrealistic megalomanic beliefs, hallucinations, and wish fulfilling delusions and employing sustained feelings of delusional superiority or entitlement.

IMMATURE DEFENSES

Defenses commonly used by adolescents are commonly seen in depression, obsessions and compulsions).

Projection: In this defense, the person attributes his unacceptable feelings/desires/deficiencies to the external world. A well-known proverb exemplifies this "A bad workman quarrels with his tools".

Somatization: In this form of defense, the conflicts are expressed in the form of bodily symptoms instead of being experienced psychologically. This kind of defense is understandable form of the saying "The pain of the mind is worse than the pain of the body". In our country especially, bodily manifestation of psychological problems is a common presentation.

Acting out: The direct expression of an unconscious wish or impulse in action is to avoid being conscious of the accompanying affect. The unconscious fantasy, involving objects, is lived out impulsively in behavior, thus gratifying the impulse more than the prohibition against it (Example is destruction of property in a fit of rage).

Hypochondriasis: The unconscious transformation of unacceptable impulses (bereavement, loneliness, or unacceptable aggressive impulses) into inappropriate somatic concern (complaints of pain, somatic illness, and neurasthenia). Existent illness may also be overemphasized or exaggerated for its evasive and regressive possibilities.

Regression: A return to a previous more comfortable and less stressful stage of behavior or functioning, to avoid the anxieties or hostilities involved in later stages. A return to earlier points of fixation is often the result of a disruption of equilibrium at a later phase of development. Example is a child who is weaned returns to drinking from a bottle during hospitalization.

Turning against the self: Changing an unacceptable impulse that is aimed at others by redirecting it against oneself, resulting in lowered self esteem, self criticism and some time injury to self (As seen in deliberate self harm, suicide).

NEUROTIC DEFENSE

(Defenses commonly seen in adults under stress and neurotic disorder patients)

Rationalization: The conflicts associated with unfulfilled needs or deficiencies are reduced by justifying statements. Another well known tale illustrates the point: "The fox which could not reach for the grapes went away saying, 'chi, these grapes are sour'."

Disassociation: In this defense there is a temporary but drastic modification of character or personal identities to avoid emotional distress.

Conversion: The conflict resolution occurs through the development of a bodily symptom which resembles a physical illness. A variety of manifestation like-tremors, paralysis, hiccups, hyperventilation, gait disturbance, abnormal body posture or movements occur. Since the symptoms occur to reduce mental tension, the person often displays indifference towards the physical manifestation. This is called as 'la belle indifference'. Sometimes the bodily symptoms may be a symbolic representation of the conflict. For example. A mother who feels guilty at having slapped her child in a fit of anger might develop a 'paralysis' of the hand.

Displacement: In this defense, the unpleasant emotional feeling like anger or anxiety are transferred to another non-threatening object when direct expression of these feelings are unacceptable. This is commonly seen in phobia and obsessive compulsive disorders. For example–A person who has a confrontation at his place of employment goes home and argues with his family.

Intellectualization: The control of affects and impulses by way of thinking about them (logic) instead of experiencing them. It is a systematic excess of thinking, deprived of its affect, to defend against anxiety caused by unacceptable impulses.

Isolation: The intrapsychic splitting or separation of the idea of an unconscious impulse from its appropriate affect, thus allowing only the idea and not the associated affect to enter awareness.

Undoing: Unconsciously motivated acts which symbolically counteract unacceptable thoughts, impulses or acts. (examples are checking of lock, frequent washing of hands etc.).

Suppression: The conscious or semiconscious decision to postpone attention to a conscious impulse or conflict.

Reaction formation: The management of unacceptable impulses by permitting expression of the impulse in antithetical form. This is equivalently an expression of the impulse in the negative. Where instinctual conflict is persistent, reaction formation can become a character trait on a permanent basis, usually as an aspect of obsessional character.

Repression: Conscious distancing of events or thoughts that are too painful or unacceptable to one's ego into the unconscious level. These feelings can continue to influence behavior in adult years if unresolved. Example is a person who was sexually abused as a child is unable to achieve a meaningful intimate relationship as an adult.

MATURE DEFENSES

(Defenses which are commonly used by psychologically and physically healthy adults with well adjusted life)

Altruism: The vicarious but constructive and instinctually gratifying services to others. This must be distinguished from altruistic surrender, which involves surrender of direct gratification or of instinctual needs in favor of fulfilling the needs of others to the detriment of the self, with vicarious satisfaction only being gained through introjection.

Anticipation: the realistic anticipation of or planning for future unpleasurable events: implies overly concerned planning, worrying, and anticipation of dire and dreadful possible outcomes. Anticipation is a common phenomenon seen in all intelligent persons.

Asceticism: In this defense, the pleasurable aspects of a desire are eliminated and gratification is derived by renunciation. This defense is illustrated by the saying of Buddha that desire is the cause of unhappiness and the means of overcoming this is to get rid of the desire.

Humor: The unacceptable or distressing feelings are expressed without personal discomfort or unpleasant effects on others. We often see this in newspapers and magazine in the form of cartoons and jokes. For example, the painful awareness about inflation may be converted into a joke "What goes up and never comes down?"—"The cost of living".

Sublimation: The wishes/impulses that are unacceptable are expressed through socially acceptable outlets (Channelization of negative impulses into creative activities). For example, a person with aggressive impulses becomes a sportsman or joins the military service.

KEY POINTS

- Defense mechanisms are mental processes which are generally unconscious and which serve the purpose of protecting the individual from anxiety generated by intrapsychic conflicts.
- Defense mechanisms are also known as Coping Mechanism.
- Patients with psychotic illness having disorders of affect, thought, and perception commonly use various defense mechanism like projection, denial, distortion, regression and turning against self.
- Patients with Neurotic disorders use commonly the Defense Mechanisms of conversion, displacement, dissociation, isolation, reaction formation and repression.
- Narcissistic Defenses are used by children and psychotics.
- Immature Defenses are commonly used by adolescents and are commonly seen in depression, obsessions and compulsions.
- Neurotic Defenses commonly seen in adults under stress and patients of neurotic disorder.
- Mature Defenses are commonly used by psychologically and physically healthy adults with well adjusted life.

5 Causes of Mental Disorders

It is difficult to pin-point exact etiology of most psychiatric disorders. Multiple factors appear to play a role in the genesis of psychiatric disorders, and it is usually a combination of factors, which may be accompanied by a precipitating stressful event that results in an illness. The contribution made by various factors may vary in different psychiatric disorders, but the etiology is multi-factorial most of the times. Schizophrenia is the most studied illness in this regard.

The different etiological factors known to cause psychiatric disorders can be grouped under genetic, familial, organic, sociological, environmental and psychological factors.

1. GENETIC FACTORS

Genetic contribution to psychiatric disorders is now a well-proven fact. The evidences accumulated from twin, adoption and family studies suggested this fact. Twin studies have provided definite evidence of role of genetic factors in etiology of schizophrenia, mood disorders and panic disorders by showing a much higher concordance rate for the respective disorders in monozygotic twins as compared with dizygotic twins. Further evidence has been provided by adoption studies where the biological offspring of schizophrenic parents reared by normal parents were shown to have higher rates of schizophrenia than the adopted offspring of normal parents, brought up by schizophrenic parents. It shows that it is the genetic contribution rather than the environmental stress of being brought up by parents having schizophrenia, that results in the increased risk of developing illness in the biological offspring's of schizophrenic parents. The family risk studies have also supported the genetic causation for schizophrenia, mood disorders, panic disorders, obsessive compulsive disorder, somatization disorder and alcohol dependence by showing an increased risk to develop the respective illness in the first degree relative compared with that in normal population.

2. ORGANIC FACTORS

Brain is the centre of functioning of mind and is the seat of control of human behavior. Thinking, decision making, memory, intelligence, emotions, control over one's behavior and awareness of surroundings are all different functions of mind. Anything which affects brain directly or indirectly can lead to disturbance in functioning of mind or behavior. Thus, brain insult due to any cause, such as trauma, infections, anoxia, vascular insufficiency, metabolic disturbances or any other pathology in brain which may be primary or secondary to a systematic cause, can lead to clinical picture resembling schizophrenia, mood disorder, anxiety disorder, personality changes or non-specific psychiatric symptoms. The detail of each functioning area of the brain has discussed separately in Chapter 2.

Brain damage occurring before birth or in early childhood may produce mental retardation or may make the child more vulnerable to childhood behavior disorders. Brain insult occurring in perinatal period due to any cause has been found to be associated with increased vulnerability to develop schizophrenia in adulthood. Degenerative changes in brain, occurring due to any cause, can lead to dementia.

3. PSYCHOLOGICAL FACTORS

Psychological factors start influencing an individual from birth onwards and continue their influence in the later life. The mother, the father, sibling and other significant people in life have effect on the individual's psychological development, and disturbance at any stage may result in increased vulnerability to develop different psychiatric disorders, depending on the stage involved and type and severity of the disturbance. For example, the crucial defect in schizophrenia is a disturbance in ego organization, which affects the interpretation of reality and the control of inner drives, such as sex and aggression. The disturbance occurs as a consequence of distortion in reciprocal relationship between the infant and the mother.

It is postulated that in schizophrenia the symptoms have symbolic meanings to patient. Depression is taught to be a result of loss of loved object. Separation from parents in childhood has been postulated to predispose to depression. Certain personality types such as oral dependant, obsessive compulsive and hysterical are probably associated with increased risk of developing depression. Panic attacks are described as an unsuccessful defense against anxiety provoking situations.

Marital disharmony in parents, broken homes, alcoholism in parents, etc. all predispose to development of psychiatric disorder at a later stage, by affecting the psychological development. Certain disorders such as phobias, panic are hypothesized to be learned behaviors, learned by the principle of conditioning.

4. PHYSIOLOGICAL FACTORS

The normal physiological variations in the body or physiological changes occurring in response to some external event such as an acute stress may also have some etiological significance. Premenstrual tension occurring in the late luteal phase in women, pregnancy and puerperium related psychological disturbances, and menopausal syndrome are examples of psychiatric syndromes accompanying various normal physiological events.

Anxiety as such is also accompanied by so many physiological changes. Metabolic changes occurring after surgery and otherwise is often responsible for delirium.

Physical deprivations like malnutrition, sleep deprivation also affect physical and mental health of an individual and may cause a number of psychiatric conditions including mental retardation, anxiety disorder, depression and other psychological conditions.

5. LIFE EVENTS AND ENVIRONMENTAL FACTORS

Stress can be caused by any factor mentioned here. Stressful life events have been found to be more common in the period immediately preceding the development of anxiety, depression, schizophrenia and other psychiatric disorders. For instance, failure in exams, failure in love, unemployment, death of near one, marital disharmony, divorce, loss of money or property are few example of stress. Chronically stressful environment can have a causative effect as well as it can delay recovery from different psychiatric disorders. Hostile and critical family environment has been found to be associated with increased risk of relapse in schizophrenia.

6. SOCIOLOGICAL FACTORS

Number of social phenomena like immigration, social changes, unemployment, violence, wars and natural disasters by their social consequences, are followed by increased risk of various psychiatric disorders such as stress reaction, adjustment disorder, anxiety disorder, depression, post traumatic stress disorder and psychotic phenomenon.

War and violence due to various reasons have great impact on mental health of an individual and predispose him to mental health problems. Similarly natural disasters like earth quakes and, floods also predispose to many abnormal behavior. Lack of social relationship and decreased social support are associated with development of depression and anxiety disorders. The braking of joint family system leading to disruption of social support is important risk factor which is likely to increase the prevalence of depression and various neurotic disorders in India in the coming years.

When it was noticed that there was concentration of schizophrenics in the congested central localities and slums in big cities, it was hypothesized that such environmental conditions play a causative role of schizophrenia **(social causation hypothesis of schizophrenia).** But now it has been well documented that the patients with schizophrenia gradually drift down in their socioeconomic and occupational status and reach places **(social drift hypothesis of schizophrenia).**

7. FAMILIAL FACTORS

The proponents of familial causation of psychiatric disorders say that there is something wrong in the family, parental upbringing, learning from family members or in family dynamics, which predisposes to a psychiatric illness. The pathological relationships or patterns of communication with in the family may lead to eventual development of schizophrenia. Familial factors also appear to play a role in etiology of phobic, somatization and somatoform pain disorders. The family environment can transfer specific phobic attitudes and behaviors to the growing child. In a similar way, the parental tendency to somatize stress may get transferred by learning to the children.

Maternal deprivation (Deprivation of child from mother's care and warmth) is bound to affect child growth. This deprivation may be due to death of mother or absence of mother at home. This predisposes to number of conditions with abnormal behavior in children.

Similarly children of disrupted families and/or broken homes go through a lot of stress and develop a delinquent behavior. Lack of discipline in children also predisposes to aggressiveness and antisocial behaviors.

SUMMARY

A combination of various etiological factors results in vulnerability in an individual to develop a psychiatric illness. Each individual has an innate psychological and biological strength to face various life stresses. Experiencing stress beyond the individual's capacity and increased vulnerability to develop an illness result in occurrence of the particular disorder.

KEY POINTS

- Identification of one cause is difficult, multiple factors appear to play a role in the genesis of psychiatric disorders.
- The different etiological factors known to cause psychiatric disorders can be grouped under genetic, familial, organic, psychological, sociological, environmental and physical factors.
- Genetic contribution to psychiatric disorders is now a well-proven fact.
- Twin studies provide definite evidence of role of genetic factors in etiology of schizophrenia, mood disorders and panic disorders by showing a much higher concordance rate for the respective disorders in monozygotic twins than dizygotic twins.
- Pathological family patterns, faulty parent-child relationship, maternal deprivation, broken homes, lack of discipline in children predisposes to delinquent behavior, aggressiveness, antisocial behaviors and number of conditions with abnormal behavior.
- Brain insult due to any cause, such as trauma, infections, anoxia, vascular insufficiency, metabolic disturbances or any other pathology can lead to clinical picture resembling schizophrenia, mood disorder, anxiety disorder, personality changes or non-specific psychiatric symptoms.
- Psychological factors start influencing an individual from birth onwards and continue their influence in the later life.
- Social phenomena like immigration, unemployment, violence, wars and natural disasters and social changes by their social consequences increase the risk of various psychiatric disorders such as stress reaction, adjustment disorder, anxiety disorder, depression, post traumatic stress disorder and psychotic phenomenon.
- Stressful life events like failure in exams, failure in love, unemployment, death of near one, marital disharmony, divorce, loss of money or property are found to be more common in the period immediately preceding the development of anxiety, depression, schizophrenia and other psychiatric disorders.
- Premenstrual tension occurring in the late luteal phase in women, pregnancy and puerperium related psychological disturbances, and menopausal syndrome are examples of psychiatric syndromes accompanying various normal physiological events.
- A combination of various etiological factors result in vulnerability in an individual to develop a psychiatric illness.

6 Understanding Stress, Conflict and Crisis

Emotional problems and minor psychiatric disorders like neurosis are frequently related to several psychological and social factors. These could be in the form of various external pressures (***stress, crisis***), internal pressure (***conflicts***), or because of faulty learning.

As human beings, we are exposed to a number of events in our lives. Some of these life events are undesirable. These undesirable events produce a mental disequilibrium in us, necessitating adjustment.

These various life events could be classified as follows:

1. **Family and social:** Interpersonal problems within the family, troubles with neighbors, son/daughter leaving home, illnesses in family members, alcoholism in a relative, interpersonal problems with in-laws, role conflicts etc.
2. **Work:** Unemployment, overwork, suspension, dismissal, transfer, trouble with colleagues, failure to get promotion, dissatisfaction with the type of work and dissatisfaction with remuneration.
3. **Financial:** Financial loss, loss of crops, large loans, difficulty in maintaining the family due to inadequate income.
4. **Marital and sexual:** Marital dissatisfaction, separation, divorce, extra-marital relationships, problems related to dowry and sexual problems.
5. **Health:** Illnesses which are life threatening like cancer, myocardial infarction; illnesses which produce disability like fractures and dislocations, congestive cardiac failure, chronic obstructive airway disease; and illnesses which are perceived as a stigma, like leprosy, AIDS etc.
6. **Education:** Inability to pursue the desired educational course, difficulty in coping with studies, failure in examinations.
7. **Bereavement:** Death of spouse, parent, child, close relative or friend.
8. **Personal:** Failure to fulfill ambitions, disappointment in love etc.
9. **Legal:** Legal disputes, violation of law, detention in jail.
10. **Migration:** Change of residence in another city, state or country.

STRESS

Stress is defined as a condition that results when a threat or challenge to one's well being requires a person to adjust. As human beings we experience number of stresses in our lives. There are two kinds of stresses:

A. *Eustress:* It is positive and motivating, as shown by one's confidence in the ability to master a challenge or stressor. This type of stress may actually enhance the feeling of well-being.

B. *Distress:* it is negative emotion and demands an exhausting type of energy, occurs in response to threat or challenge.

Stress is further defined in term of acute and chronic stress. Acute stress constitutes the reaction to an immediate threat, commonly called the "fight or flight" response. Chronic stress occurs, when the situation is ongoing or continuous, such as chronic illness of family members.

Sign and Symptoms of Stress

Common symptoms of stress generally fall in four categories:

1. **Physical symptoms:** Physical symptoms are usually triggered by arousal of autonomic nervous system and include increase in heart rate and blood pressure, faster breathing, abdominal cramping, nausea, vomiting, muscles ache, headache and insomnia.
2. **Psychological symptoms:** It includes lack of concentration, loss of memory, inability to make decision, forgetfulness and confusion.
3. **Emotional symptoms:** Emotional responses may include anxiety, nervousness, frustration, anger, irritability and excessive worry.
4. **Behavioral symptoms:** Impact of stress also affects behavior and present as pacing, fidgety movements, nail biting, smoking, drinking and throwing things.

Management of Stress

What do people do when faced with such stress factors? People employ several strategies called coping mechanisms to deal with their difficulties. In other words coping mechanisms are conscious mental or behavioral strategies that are adopted by people to tackle stressors. Coping mechanisms can be healthy or unhealthy.

Coping strategies generally fall in four categories:

- **Adaptive:** When the problem is solved in a rational and productive way and anxiety is reduced, it is said to be adaptive.
- **Palliative:** If the solution temporarily relieves anxiety and problems still exist and must be dealt with again at a latter time, it is termed as palliative.
- **Maladaptive:** If unsuccessful attempts are being made to decrease the anxiety without attempting to solve the problems, these are maladaptive coping strategies.
- **Dysfunctional:** The individual does not attempt to reduce the anxiety or solve the problems. This is considered dysfunctional management.

Stress is a part of life. We have choices to replace negative feelings with more positive ones. We can stand back and look realistically at the situation. The outcome is rarely as bad as we fear. Coping strategies are learned by observation of those who model them in our family and social environment. These can be either adaptive or maladaptive. Nurses have a major role in helping patients with stress to cope more effectively. Some of the techniques for managing stress are as follows:

A. **Strategies aimed at resolution of the problem**

1. **Problem solving techniques:** This consists of the following steps (a) Evaluation of the problem or problems in terms of their magnitude and the existing resources to deal with the same (b) Formulating alternative solutions (c) Choosing the appropriate solution (d) Applying the appropriate solution to examine its effectiveness.
2. **Discussion with family members and friends:** A better understanding of the problem and the possible solutions is achieved by discussion with family members and friends. Further they can provide adequate support to the patient to enable him to overcome the crisis situation.
3. **Consulting an expert adviser or counsellor:** When a stressor is of such a

nature that problem solving techniques generated by the patient and support from the family members fail to be effective, often an expert adviser, for example the village leader or counselor may enable the subject to deal with his difficulties.

B. **Strategies aimed at minimizing the effect of the stress factor**

1. **Change of environment:** Sometimes a change of environment brings down the distress produced by a chronic stress and provides the person with enough strength to deal with his problem.
2. **Physical activity:** Many individuals engage in physical activities as a form of diversion from their worries. Involving oneself in work, physical exercises, and sports are some of the common strategies employed by people.
3. **Mental activity:** Mental activity is another form of diversion. Activities like reading, writing, listening to music and meditation are helpful.
4. **Visiting places of worship:** Some people derive solace from visiting places of worship. Faith sustains the individual's strength to deal with his difficulties.
5. **Seeking support from others:** Other people in social environment like family members and friends may provide the needed support to the patient. Social welfare organizations, religious organizations and voluntary agencies are frequently helpful.
6. **Psychological acceptance:** Often people learn to accept an inevitable situation by comparing their difficulties with those of others–"After all, my troubles are much less compared to his". Others may attribute their difficulties to Karma of Fate –"What is destined will occur". Some way even looks at the positive effect of the stressors–"Every event is an experience to me and I shall learn from it".

While these are healthy mechanisms to deal with stressors, other may use unhealthy means of dealing with them. Some may avoid all forms of difficulties. Some individuals become excessively dependent on others. Others may start abusing drugs.

In general, people cope with stress factor better if the stress is single, of a mild nature, if similar stress has been experienced earlier, if adequate preparation has occurred to deal with the stressor, and when support from others is available. Emotional problems result when people cannot cope with the stressors or where they use faulty methods of coping.

Illustrative case history: Mr. Krishan, a 43-year-old male, working as a school teacher came for consultation with symptoms of tiredness, palpitations and sleep disturbance, of 2 months duration. On interview he reported experiencing symptoms of anxiety and depression. During subsequent enquiry, it was evident that a number of undesirable events had occurred in his life and had caused his emotional problems. His wife had been suffering from attacks of migraine since several years which had increased in frequency and intensity. Three months prior to his present consultation, he was diagnosed to be suffering from diabetes mellitus. As a consequence patient became apprehensive as to whether he would develop a life threatening complication of the illness. A week after the diagnosis of diabetes mellitus, his son met with a road accident and sustained a fracture. Ten days prior to his consultation, his brother was suspended from his job, apparently because of financial mismanagement. Patient reported being very upset as a result of all these incidents.

The above case history clearly illustrates how recent life events precipitate an emotional disturbance.

CONFLICTS

In the previous section we noted that a number of environmental stress factor (external pressure) could produce emotional disturbance. Emotional disturbance can also be the result of conflicts (internal pressure).

What do we mean by the term conflict? As human beings we experience various needs, deficiencies and desires from time to time. Sometimes we become aware of these needs/deficiencies/desires so strongly that we seek to fulfill them immediately. If there is any hindrance to the fulfillment of these needs, then we experience a conflict or mental struggle. Such conflicts can also arise when we are faced with two opposing needs and we have to choose between the two. The following examples in box illustrate the nature of conflict.

> **Example 1:** An employee working in his home town gets a promotion cum transfer. If he accepts the transfer, he has to move away from his town leaving his aged parents, wife and children. If he remains in his home town he gets no promotion. This results in a conflict.
> **Example 2:** A student has a strong desire to become an engineer. However, his parents to whom he has great regard always wanted him to become a doctor. Having to choose between these two alternative produces a conflict.

How is conflict dealt with? There are certain processes called defense mechanisms which serve to reduce the tension produced by the conflicts. These are mental processes of which we are generally unconscious and which serve to reduce the mental disturbance produced by the conflicts.

The following are examples of some defense mechanisms:

1. **Denial:** The existence of something that can induce a conflict is denied. For example, we often read about accidents/deaths etc. but we use defense of denial to prevent the painful awareness of reality that these things can occur to ourselves. The use of denial as a defense can be noticed in persons with alcoholism, who often state the consumption of alcohol has never been a problem to them. Similarly, the initial reaction to the diagnosis of a threatening illness like cancer is one of denial.
2. **Projection:** In this defense, the person attributes his unacceptable feelings/desires/deficiencies to the external world. A well known proverb exemplifies this "A bad workman quarrels with his tools".
3. **Rationalization:** The conflicts associated with unmet needs or deficiencies are reduced by justifying statements. Another well known tale illustrates the point: 'The fox who could not reach the grapes went away saying "these grapes are sour" '.
4. **Somatization:** In this form of defense, the conflicts are expressed in the form of bodily symptoms instead of being experienced psychologically. This kind of defense is understandable from the saying "The pain of the mind is worse than the pain of body". In our country especially, bodily manifestation of psychological problems is a common presentation.
5. **Dissociation:** In this defense, there is temporary but drastic modification of character or personal identity to avoid emotional distress. See an example in box.

> Ms. Rani, a young woman of rural background was reported to be possessed by evil spirits. During these attacks of possession, Rani personal appearance would become dishevelled, and her voice, louder. She would claim that she is the spirit of Savita, her friend, who had died 6

months ago. These possession attacks would last about 15-minute to half an hour each time, after which Rani would have no knowledge of what occurred during these episodes. During one of these episodes the 'spirit of Savita suddenly warned Krishna, Rani's husband, and Maya, her mother-in-law to stop ill-treating Rani, failing which they would face dire consequences. Following this there was an improvement in the relationships in Rani's family.

The above case history illustrates how Rani's conflict was resolved through possession attacks, which are culturally accepted dissociative states.

6. **Conversion:** The conflict resolution occurs through the development of a bodily symptom which resembles a physical illness. A variety of manifestations like tremors, paralysis, hiccups, hyperventilation, gait disturbances, abnormal body posture or movements occur. Since the symptoms occur to reduce mental tension, the person often displays indifference towards the physical manifestation. This is called 'la belle indifference'. Sometimes the bodily symptoms may be a symbolic representation of the conflict. For example, a mother who feels guilty of slapping her child in a fit of anger might develop a paralysis of the hand.
7. **Displacement:** In this defense, the unpleasant emotional feelings like anger or anxiety are transferred to another non-threatening object when direct expressions of these feelings are unacceptable.

   Example: A 45-year-old engineer presented with history suggestive of anxiety neurosis of several years duration. One of his main problems was his frequent angry outbursts at his secretary. On further enquiry, it was evident that patient had strained relationship with his wife. The anger at his wife was being displaced on to his secretary.
8. **Asceticism:** In this defense, the pleasurable aspects of a desire are eliminated and gratification is derived by renunciation. This defense is illustrated by the saying of Buddha that desire is the cause of unhappiness and the means of overcoming this to get rid of the desire.
9. **Humour:** The unacceptable or distressing feelings are expressed without personal discomfort or unpleasant effect on others. We often see this in newspapers and magazines in the form of cartoons and jokes. For example, the painful awareness about inflation may be converted into a joke "What goes up and never comes down?" "The cost of living!"
10. **Sublimation:** The wishes/impulses which are unacceptable are expressed through socially acceptable outlets. For example, a person with aggressive impulses becomes a sportsman or joins the military services.

It is important to note that these defense mechanisms are generally "unconscious". That is, we are not generally aware of the operation of these mechanisms in our day to day life. They are not always pathological. To a certain extent they are normal phenomena and are employed by all of us at different times. Some defenses like asceticism, humor or sublimation are classified as mature defenses. People employing these defenses make a healthy adjustment and do not develop emotional problems. Emotional problems arise because the conflicts are so severe that the defenses are ineffective. Mental disorders result when unhealthy defenses are used or healthy defenses breakdown.

Exploration of conflict/stress factor

Identification of conflict or stress factor is an art, which includes following steps:

1. Assure—**Confidentiality.**
2. Establish **Rapport.**
3. Ask **Open ended questions.**
4. Enquire **Specifically about stress factor.**
5. Involve **Significant others.**

CRISIS

In 1961, psychiatrist Gerald Caplan defined a crisis as occurring when a person faces a problem that can not be solved by customary problem solving methods. When the usual problem solving methods no longer work, a person's life balance or equilibrium is upset. During the period of disequilibrium there is rise in inner tension and anxiety, followed by emotional upset. Usually crisis occurs when the precipitating stressful event is unusual or rare. The state of dysfunction is usually receptive to the right intervention that can help the person stabilize and regain a sense of power and control over their being.

Many life events can evoke a crisis. Obvious crisis evoking events includes natural and manmade disasters (flood, fires, earthquakes, wars, bombing etc.), trauma (rape, sexual abuse, assaults), interpersonal crisis (divorce, marriage, birth of child).

Crisis Response

The crisis response is similar in all theses different situations. First, an event occurs that is perceived by a person as a threat and for which the usual coping methods do not work. Tension builds, and the person attempts to adapt to the situation by using new coping techniques that emerge naturally or are supported by helpers. If adaptation occurs, the person is able to cope with future threatening events. If the person cannot cope, overall functioning decreases, and the person does not return to the previous level of functioning. When these measures do not reduce anxiety, anxiety can overwhelm the person and lead to serious personality disorganizations, fear, violence or suicidal behavior which signals the person is in crisis.

Crisis Intervention

- The state of crisis is intolerable for more than a few weeks if help is not received. The dysfunctional state that continues without resolving the underlying problem will result in physical or mental symptoms.
- The outcome depends on the actions taken by the individual to cope with the crisis and those taken by others to intervene. During a crisis, an individual is often more receptive to support from others and can learn adaptive coping strategies to assist in the resolution.
- Crisis intervention deals with the present situation and resolution of the immediate issue. Early intervention in assisting the individual to manage the current situation promotes the best chance for a positive outcome. Once the anxiety level is reduced to a tolerable level, the individual can be assisted in defining the problem, determining available support, and setting realistic goals for resolution of the issue.
- The nurse is integral in providing support and returning control to the patient. Listening to what the patient says both verbally and non-verbally gives insight into the problem. This allows the nurse to help the patient identify alternative ways of reducing anxiety and feeling of powerlessness.
- If person is suicidal, protective measures must be initiated to provide a feeling of safety and security.
- Outcome is to be aimed at promoting optimum psychological and physiological functioning.

KEY POINTS

- Stress is defined as a condition that results when a threat or challenge to one's well-being requires a person to adjust.
- Stress are of two type—Eustress—(positive and motivating) and Distress (negative emotion and demands an exhausting type of energy).
- Common symptoms of stress generally fall in four categories: (i) Physical **Symptoms** like increase in heart rate and blood pressure, faster breathing, abdominal cramping, nausea, vomiting, muscles ache, headache etc. (ii) Psychological **Symptoms** like lack of concentration, loss of memory, inability to make decision, forgetfulness and confusion. (iii) Emotional **Symptoms** including anxiety, nervousness, frustration, anger, irritability and excessive worry, and (iv) Behavioral **Symptoms** presented as pacing, fidgety movements, nail biting, smoking, drinking and throwing things.
- Coping mechanisms are adopted by people to tackle stressors. Coping mechanisms can be healthy or unhealthy and generally fall in four categories. **Adaptive, Palliative, Maladaptive, and Dysfunctional.**
- Conflicts can arise when we are faced with two opposing needs and we have to choose between the two.
- Defense mechanisms are mental processes, which are generally unconscious and which serve to reduce the mental disturbance produced by the conflicts.
- Identification of conflict or stress factor is an art, which includes following steps: Confidentiality, Rapport, Open ended questions, Enquiry about Specific stress factor and Involvement of Significant others.
- Crisis is a condition occurring when a person faces a problem that can not be solved by customary problem solving methods.
- When the usual problem solving methods no longer work, a person's life balance or equilibrium is upset and there is rise in inner tension and anxiety, followed by emotional upset.
- The state of crisis is intolerable for more than a few weeks if help is not received.
- Early intervention in assisting the individual to manage the current situation promotes the best chance for a positive outcome.
- The nurse is integral in providing support and returning control to the patient. Listening to what the patient says both verbally and nonverbally gives insight into the problem.
- In case of crisis, if person is suicidal, protective measures must be initiated to provide a feeling of safety and security.

7 Common Signs and Symptoms in Psychiatry

Psychiatric disorders result in abnormalities affecting the patient's appearance, behavior, thinking, mood, perception, volition, attention, concentration, orientation, memory and judgement. Eliciting abnormalities in these areas are essential in arriving at a psychiatric diagnosis.

1. DISORDERS OF PERCEPTION

These can be considered under following categories:

a. **Sensory distortions: Sensory distortions may occur in any modality. Mainly they are of two types i.e. change in intensity and change in quality.**

   Change in intensity

   Hyperaesthesia—Increase intensity of sensation.

   Hypoaesthesia—Decrease intensity of sensation.

   Change in quality

   Consumption of some drugs and toxic substances are liable to produce these changes like Yellow vision with santonin or metallic taste in mouth with metronidazole.

b. **Sensory deceptions:**

   Illusion–Stimuli from perceived object are combined with a mental image to produce false perception. e.g. Perceiving rope as snake, while looking into mirror instead of seeing his own head he sees the head of a pig.

   Hallucination–A false perception in absence of external stimuli of sensory modality involved. Types of hallucinations are:

   - **Auditory Hallucination**–Schizophrenia, OMD and Severe Depression.
   - **Visual Hallucination**–Acute Organic state, Epilepsy, Temporal lobe epilepsy (TLE) and Drug dependence.
   - **Olfactory Hallucination** (Hallucination of smell)–TLE, Schizophrenia.
   - **Tactile Hallucination** (Hallucination of touch)– Cocaine, Schizophrenia.
   - **Somatic Hallucination** (Hallucinations of bodily sensations)–Hallucinations occurring while a person is falling asleep are called hypnagogic hallucinations and those occurring while a person is awakening from sleep are called hypnopompic hallucinations.

c. **Abnormal experience of self and environment:**

   Depersonalization–A subjective sense of being strange, unreal or unfamiliar about oneself.

   Derealization–The subjective sense of the environment being strange or unreal.

2. DISORDERS OF THOUGHT

Thinking is the most important function of human mind. Abnormalities of thinking have an important

part in diagnosis of these disorders. It is customary to classify thought disorders into 4 types:
- Disorders of stream of thought.
- Disorder of form of thought.
- Disorder of possession of thought.
- Disorder of content of thought.

A. Disorders of stream of thought

Pressure of speech: Characterized by an increase in the quantity of spontaneous speech. Patient talks rapidly and it is difficult to interrupt him. Even when interrupted, he often continues to talk. Speech tends to be loud and emphatic.
Poverty of speech: Spontaneous speech restricted. Replies to questions tend to be brief and unelaborated. Replies may be monosyllabic and some question left unanswered altogether.
Dysarthria: Difficulty in articulation but not in choice of words or content.

B. Disorders of form of thought

Loosening of association: The lack of adequate logical linkages between two consecutive thoughts is known as loosening of associations. when severe, it can make speech incoherent.
Derailment: Gradual or sudden deviation in train of thought as evident in spontaneous speech, sometimes used synonymously with loosening of association.
Tangentiality: Patient tends to wander away from the intended point, moving further and further away, never returning to the original idea.
Incoherence: The speech is essentially un-understandable because words and phrases are stringed together without any logical connection, disregarding rules of grammar. Sometimes referred to as word salad. It is seen in schizophrenia.
Neologism: New words created by the patient often combining syllables from existing words. Though not understandable to others, the patient may have his own meaning for these words.
Clang association: Use of words which sound similar but not related in meaning. May lead to rhyming and punning and often seen in manic patients.
Echolalia: Patient echoes or repeats the word or phrase of the interviewer.
Flight of Idea: Rapid succession of fragmentary thought or speech. The contents change abruptly and may be incoherent without loosing logical connection.
Retardation of thought: The train of thought is slow down and number of ideas and mental images, which present themselves, is decreased.
Circumstantiality: Here thinking proceeds slowly with many unnecessary trivial details, but finally the point is reached. It is often seen in Schizophrenia, epileptic personality changes.
Perseveration: Pathological stimulation of same response to different stimuli, as in a repetition of same verbal response to different questions. Seen in OMD, Schizophrenia etc.
Verbigeration: Meaningless and stereotyped repetition of words or phrases over and over again.
Thought blocking: Sudden arrest of train of thought, leaving a blank. An entirely new thought may then begin.

C. Disorders of possession of thought

Obsession: Stereotyped, Recurrent, persistent thoughts, Images or impulse which occur in spite of person's effort to get rid of it. When it occurs he realizes that it is senseless or at least that it is dominating and persisting without cause.
Thought Alienation: Patient thinks that his thoughts are under the control of outside agency or others are participating in his thinking.
- Thought insertion (Person experiences that thoughts are imposed by some external forces on his passive mind).
- Thought Block (experiences that thoughts are blocked by some external forces).

- Thought Broadcasting (one experience that his thought is broadcast outside so that others come to know what he is thinking).
- Thought Withdrawal (thoughts are being withdrawn by an outside agency against his will).

D. Disorders of thought content

Delusion: It is a false, firm, unshakable belief of morbid origin which is out of keeping with patient's social and cultural background. The types are following:

1. **Delusion of grandeur**–Patient believe that he is an important and extraordinary person having a lot of money, power and social status and is able to help others.
2. **Delusion of persecution**–Person believes that people in environment such as members of family, neighbours, or friends are working against him and want to harm or kill him.
3. **Delusion of infidelity**–Person believes that his life partner is unfaithful to him/her. Patient always keeps strong vigilance over life partner's acts.
4. **Delusion of love**–The patients are convinced that some person is in love with them although the alleged lover himself may have never even spoken to them.
5. **Delusion of ill-health** –Patients believe that they have some incurable disease such as Cancer, Tuberculosis, Brain tumor etc.
6. **Delusion of Guilt**–Patient believes that he is the worst sinner and has not only ruined his family, but is also responsible for all the calamities in the world, and insists that he will rot in hell for this.

3. SPEECH DISORDERS

Stammering and stuttering: The normal flow of speech is interrupted by pauses or by repetition of fragments of the word.

Mutism: Complete loss of Speech. May occur in disturbed children, Hysteria, Depression, Schizophrenia and Catatonia.

Talking past the point, Vorbeireden: Contents of the patient's replies to question show that he understands what has been asked and is deliberately talking about an associated topic.

Ex. If asked:
What is the color of grass?—White.
What is the color of snow?—Green.

It is common in Hysteria, dementia and under trial criminals.

Neologism: Refers to construction of a new word or ordinary word which he uses in a special way. It is common in Schizophrenia.

Word salad: Incoherent mixture of words without sense. Patient talks utter nonsense.

4. DISORDERS OF MEMORY

Amnesia: Partial or total inability to recall past experiences, may be organic or emotional in origin.

Paramnesia: Falsification of memory by distortion of recall, like:

Confabulation: Unconscious filling of gaps in memory by imagined experiences that patient believes but that have no basis in fact.

Déjà vu: An illusion of visual recognition in which a new situation is incorrectly regarded as a repetition of a previous memory.

Deja entendu: Illusion of auditory recognition.

Jamais vu: False feeling of unfamiliarity with a situation one had experienced.

5. DISORDERS OF MOOD AND AFFECT

Mood refers to pervasive and sustained emotional reaction which is subjectively experienced and reported by the patient. Disturbances of mood include:

e.g. **Dysphoric**–An unpleasant mood.

Expansive–A high mood with an overestimation of one's significance and importance.

Irritable.

Euphoria–Mood of intense elation with feeling of grandeur.

Depressive–Feeling of sadness.

Affect–A emotional reaction at a given moment expressed by patient and observed by others.

e.g. **Inappropriate affect**—Intensity of feeling is not appropriate to the situation.

Blunted affect—A severe reduction in intensity of emotional feeling tone.

Restricted affect—A reduction in intensity of feeling, less intense than in blunted affect.

Flat affect—Total or near total absence of any sign of emotional expression.

Labile affect—Rapid and abrupt change in affect unrelated to external stimuli.

6. DISTURBANCES OF SPEECH AND COMMUNICATION

Pressure of speech: Characterized by an increase in the spontaneous speech. Patient talks rapidly and it is difficult to interrupt him. Even when interrupted, he often continues to talk. Speech tends to be loud and emphatic.

Poverty of speech: Spontaneous speech restricted. Replies to question tend to be brief and unelaborated. Replies may be monosyllabic and some question left unanswered altogether.

Dysarthria: Difficulty in articulation but not in choice of words or content.

Echolalia: Psychopathological repetition of words or phases of one person by another.

Echopraxia: A Pathological initiation of movements of one person by another.

Catalepsy: General term for an immobile position that is constantly maintained.

7. MOTOR SYMPTOMS

1. **Retardation (Slowness and under activity):** In this state person performs all activities very slowly and takes a long time to initiate them.
2. **Stupor:** Marked by slowed motor activity, often to a point of immobility and seeming unawareness of surroundings.
3. **Rigidity:** Assumption of a rigid posture, against all efforts to be moved.
4. **Posturing:** Voluntary assumption of an inappropriate or bizarre posture, generally maintained for a long period of time.
5. **Waxy flexibility:** The person can be moulded into a position which is then maintained. When the examiner moves the person's limb, he feels as if it were made of wax.
6. **Negativism:** Motiveless resistance to all attempts to be moved or to all instructions.
7. **Stereotype:** Repetitive fixed pattern of physical action or speech.
8. **Mannerisms:** Stereotyped involuntary movements.
9. **Automatism:** Automatic preference of acts representative of unconscious symbolic activity. Automatic actions and speech are seen in clear form in the catatonic form of schizophrenia.
10. **Echopraxia:** In this condition patient imitates the examiner's movement without being asked to do so.

KEY POINTS

- Psychiatric patients exhibit abnormality in appearance, behavior, thinking, mood, perception, volition, attention, concentration, orientation, memory and judgement. Eliciting abnormalities in these areas are essential in arriving at a psychiatric diagnosis.
- Illusion and Hallucinations are disorders of perception.
- Hallucinations occurring while a person is falling asleep are called hypnagogic hallucinations and those occurring while a person is awakening from sleep are called hypnopompic hallucinations.
- Thought disorders are commonly seen in schizophrenia and obsession.
- Delusion is a false, firm, unshakable belief of morbid origin which is out of keeping with patient's social and cultural background.
- "Mood" refers to pervasive and sustained emotional reaction, which is subjectively experienced and reported by patient and "Affect" is emotional reaction at a given moment experienced by patient and observed by others.
- Motor symptoms like Rigidity, posturing, waxy flexibility, Automatism are characteristic symptoms of catatonic schizophrenia.
- Déjà vu is a illusion of visual recognition in which a new situation is incorrectly regarded as a repetition of a previous memory and Jamais-vu is false feeling of unfamiliarity with a situation one had experienced.
- Flight of Idea is commonly seen in Mania.

8 Classification of Mental Disorders

The history of mental disorders is described by various authors in different ways. The various classificatory systems used in Psychiatry date back to Greek physician Hippocrates, who first rejected the idea of demonology and introduced the terms 'Mania' and 'Hysteria' as forms of mental illness in the fifth century B.C. Similarly Plato (400 B.C) also described two kinds of madness. That in which the appetitive soul lost the domination of the rational soul, and the madness inspired by the gods, "Divine Madness". In Prevedic and Vedic era too Bhuta Vidhya of Ayurveda relates to what is new Psychiatry. Similarly, 'Manas' and 'Unmand' correspond to mind and Insanity and treatment by faith healers or temple treat was in practice. Since then, each era has introduced its own psychiatric classification.

However it was only in later part of the 17th century that the mentally ill were considered worthy of human treatment. Philip Pinel (1745-1826) in France first emphasized on human approach to treatment of mentally ill persons and unchained them in 1792. This approach led to the various reforms in the management of these patients all over the world and the mentally ill were given better living conditions and started receiving kind treatment.

Psychiatric disorders have been differently classified for the last few centuries. Unfortunately psychiatric disorders have varying symptoms as well as multiple etiology, due to which classification is not very stable.

First major classification of mental illness was based on the distinction between disorders arising from disease of brain (Organic) and those with no such basis (Functional).

Organic Psychiatric Disorders are the conditions which possibly arise from diseases of brain. Examples are Dementia, Delirium and other Organic Mental Disorders.

Functional Psychiatric Disorders are those where no such basis (disease of brain) is present. Examples are Schizophrenia, Manic Depressive Psychosis, and Depression etc.

Because of greater knowledge regarding the involvement of organic factors in etiology of mental disorders, now this traditional classification is losing its significance and with advanced research and understanding in anatomy and physiology of brain, number of factors have been detected in etiology of psychiatric disorders. So we can say that now the traditional psychiatry is moving towards the biological psychiatry.

It is common dichotomy in psychiatry to divide the functional mental disease into Psychosis and Neurosis. The term 'Psychosis' refers to severe psychiatric disorder with grossly disturbed behavior, loss of contact with reality and lack of insight, whereas the Neurosis are the psychiatric disorders of lesser severity with contact of reality and present insight.

Neurosis and Psychosis

Neurosis	*Psychosis*
1. Minor Psychiatric disorders where the awareness regarding illness is present	1. Major disorders in which awareness of illness is absent
2. Touch with reality remains present	2. Touch with reality remains absent
3. Patient does not construct a false environment.	3. Patient constructs a false environment
4. No gross Impairment in thinking perception and personality of patient	4. Patients show gross impairment in thinking, perception and personality
5. Social relationship and behavior are usually not affected	5. Social relationship and behavior are markedly affected
6. Patient's judgment will be intact	6. Patient's judgment will be impaired
7. No Gross personality disintegration	7. Partial or complete personality disintegration
8. Ego dystonic	8. Ego syntonic

CURRENT CLASSIFICATORY SYSTEMS

During the last four-five decades diagnostic method in psychiatry has been standardized and new classification has been developed. The present authentic classifications are:

- **DSM (Diagnostic and Statistical Manual of mental disorder):** This is an American Psychiatric Association's classification of mental disorders and usually followed in USA, Canada and a few other countries. The DSM-IV has a multi-axial system of diagnosis, in which an individual patient is diagnosed on five separate axis. The five axis of DSM-IV are:
  - I. Clinical psychiatric diagnosis.
  - II. Personality disorder and mental retardation.
  - III. General medical conditions.
  - IV. Psychosocial and environmental problems.
  - V. Global assessment of functioning.
- **ICD (International Classification of Disease by W.H.O.)**
  This is a WHO's classification for all diseases in which chapter fifth deals with mental and behavioral disorders. The current 10th edition is in practice since 1992 and is applicable all over the world except USA. In India we generally follow the ICD classification system. The broad categories of ICD-10 are as follows (for detailed classification see index).

ICD–10 Classification of Mental Disorders

ICD–10 uses an alphanumerical format. The section dealing with mental, behavioral and developmental disorders are placed under the alphabet F and grouped from 00 to 99. The major groups are:

1. **F.00-09 Organic including Symptomatic Mental Disorder**
   - Dementia
   - Delirium
   - Amnesic Syndrome
   - Other OMD.
2. **F 10-19 Mental and behavioral Disorders due to Psychoactive Substance use**
   Alcohol, opioids, cannabis, sedative, hypnotics, hallucinogens etc.
3. **F 20-29 Schizophrenia, schizotypal and delusional disorders**
4. **F 30-39 Mood (Affective) Disorders**
   - Mania
   - M.D.P.
   - Depression
   - Persistence Mood Disorders
5. **F 40-49 Neurotic, Stress related and Somatoform Disorders**
   Anxiety Disorders
   Phobia

Panic Disorders
OCD
Ac. Stress Reaction
Conversion Disorders
Dissociation Disorders
Somatization Disorders
Hypocondriacal Disorders

6. F 50-59 Behavioral Syndrome associated with Psychological disturbances and physical factors:
- Eating Disorders
- Sleeping Disorders
- Sexual Disorders

7. F 60-69 Disorder of Adult Personality and Behavior disorders
- Personality Disorders
- Impulse Disorders
- Sexual Perversion Disorders

8. F 70-79 Mental Retardation
- Mild
- Moderate
- Severe

9. F 80-89 Disorders of Psychological Development
- Reading Disorder
- Speech Disorder
- Writing Disorder
- Childhood Autism

10. F 90-99 Childhood and Adolescent Behavioral and Emotional Disorders with onset usually occurring in childhood and adolescence
- Hyper Kinetic Child
- Conduct Disorder
- Other Childhood Disorders.

KEY POINTS

- Psychiatry is a branch of medicine that deals with diagnosis, management and rehabilitation of mental disorders.
- Psychosis refers to severe psychiatric disorder with grossly disturbed behavior, loss of contact with reality and lack of insight.
- Neuroses are the psychiatric disorders of lesser severity with contact of reality and present insight.
- Organic Mental Disorders are the conditions which possibly arise from diseases of brain. Examples are Dementia, Delirium and other Organic Mental Disorders like organic Amnesic Syndrome.
- Functional Psychiatric Disorders are those where no such basis (disease of brain) is present. Examples are Schizophrenia, Manic Depressive Psychosis, Depression etc.
- Philip Pinel (1745-1826) in France first emphasized on human approach to treatment of mentally ill persons and unchained them. He is also known as father of modern psychiatry.
- ICD-10 is a International Classification of Disease given by WHO, usually followed all over the world (except USA) for classification of mental disorders.
- DSM-IV (Diagnostic and Statistical Manual of mental disorder) is an American Psychiatric Association's classification of mental disorders usually followed in USA.

9 Historical Developments in Mental Health Care

Throughout history, number of factors were believed to cause mental disorders depending on underlying popular beliefs of the times. Prehistoric healers practiced an ancient surgical technique of removing disk of bone from skull to let out the evil spirits. In early Christian period sin or demonic possessions were thought to cause mental disorders.

Later in medieval era (1000-1300), many believed that disorders were product of dysfunctional environments, and individuals were removed from their sick environment and placed in protected asylums. The first institution for the mentally ill was opened in London as **the Bethlehem Royal hospital** in 1247. The insane received cruel and inhuman treatment and were require to wear chains. During the renaissance, in early 1400s, there was a growing interest in abnormal human behavior and a early classification of mental disorders was developed by scholars and physicians. Despite of this growing interest, care given to mentally sick did not improve.

It was perhaps during the seventeenth century that conditions reached their lowest and most horrific point. Those with symptoms of insanity were locked in cells, starved, brutally beaten and neglected. In the late 1700s, psychiatry emerged as a separate division of medical science. Those connected with specialty began to question the way, those with mental problem were treated. Along with European countries, the U.S. Colonies began to open asylums to house the insane along with prisoners and orphans. It was considered a place for the rejected of the society. Care was provided by the poor and included such practices as blood-letting, purging, and confinement chairs.

The emergence of enlightened political ideas in the late 18th century led to the advent of moral treatment in mental health care, which was characterized by kindness, compassion and a pleasant environment for patients. It was during this time that **Philippe Pinel** (1745-1826), who was a French physician, believed that insanes were sick patients who needed special treatment. Once installed in his position, he ordered the removal of the chains and respectfully placed the patients under care of physicians. At about the same time ***William Tuke*** (1732-1822) of England raised funds for the same cause and founded the York Retreat hospital in London and provided humanitarian care to the patients. In 1812, ***Benzamine Rush*** referred to as the "Father of American Psychiatry" wrote the first American text book of psychiatry. Around the middle of the nineteenth century, there was a change in perspective towards the care provided to those with mental illness.

MENTAL HEALTH NURSING: HISTORICAL PERSPECTIVES

Mental health nursing encompasses identification and treatment of those problems that occur as a result of human responses to an actual or potential threat. This branch of nursing has evolved into a specialized area of practice, employing the use of various theories about human behavior and learned skills, and therapeutic interventions.

Psychiatric nursing as a profession began to emerge in the late nineteenth century, and by the twentieth century it had become speciality with unique roles and functions.

In 1873 ***Linda Richards*** graduated from the New England hospital for woman and children in Bostan. She developed better nursing care in psychiatric hospitals and organized nursing services and educational programs in the state mental hospitals in Illinosis . Several years later, she traveled to England to receive more training at St. Thomas's Hospital in London, the hospital established by Florence Nightingale in 1860. Here she met Florence Nightingale and was trained under her. For these activities, Linda Richards is called the first American Psychiatric Nurse. The first school to prepare nurses to care for the mentally ill opened at Mc Lean Hospitals in waverly, Massachusetts, in 1882. It was a two years training program with focus on patient's physical needs including nutrition, hygiene, medication etc. Until the end of nineteenth century, there was little change in the role of psychiatric nurses. One of Linda Richard's important contributions was her emphasis on assessing both physical and emotional needs of the patient.

In 1913, John Hopkins became the first School of Nursing to include a fully developed course for psychiatric nursing in the curriculum. Other schools soon followed.

Harriet Bailey wrote Nursing Mental Disease, the first psychiatric nursing text book in1920.

Political and social changes of twentieth century were beginning to influence the present and future roles of psychiatric nurses. Although most patients with mental illness were still institutionalized in state mental hospitals, there was a growing trend toward the provision of community based treatment at inpatient hospital units that specialized in the care of mental illness. This meant growing need for trained nurses to fill both new and expanded roles. By the 1950s, many steps were taken towards improved conditions and treatment methods. The expanded philosophy of mental health nursing was based on the scientific and systematic approach, later referred as nursing process.

The work of Hildegard Peplau (1909-1999) laid the groundwork for interpersonal and interactive processes in nurse patient relationship. Peplau believed that nurse acts as a resource person, counselor, role model and support person for the patient.

It was during this period that the first psychotherapeutic drugs were introduced. These drugs provided relief of symptoms and put an end to the need for physical restraint in straight-jackets and for lobotomies to remove portion of the brain to control behaviors. Sedatives were developed that quieted clients. Shortly thereafter, antidepressant and anti anxiety drugs were developed. These developments allowed practitioners to control the symptoms of mental illness without restrain and other induced methods. Gradually, as these changes occurred, the political climate changed and legislation was passed to make care of the mentally ill mandatory, available, and standardized.

As this new era of treatment emerged, the movement to deinstitutionalize patients with mental illness was in motion. Between 1950 and 1980 the number of institutionalized clients dropped considerably and a need for community based mental health care gained momentum. Nurses can and will continue to play a part in addressing the needs of the mentally ill and their families. The interpersonal therapeutic relationship between the nurse and the patient is perhaps the most fundamental of healing arts.

IMPORTANT LANDMARKS IN MENTAL HEALTH NURSING

Year	Contribution
1247	First institution for mentally ill was opened in London as Bethlehem Royal Hospital.
1812	Benzamin Rush referred to as the "Father of American Psychiatry", wrote the first American textbook of Psychiatry.
1842	Social reformer Dorothea Dix, advocated for humane treatment of patients with mental illness.
1873	Linda Richards graduated from New England Hospital for Women and Children.
1882	First school to prepare nurses to care for the mentally ill was opened at McLean Hospital, Waver by in Massachusetts.
1913	John Hopkins became the first school of nursing to include a fully developed course for psychiatric nursing in curriculum.
1952	Publication of Hildegarde E. Peplau's Interpersonal Relations in Nursing.
1954	First graduate program in Psychiatric Nursing established at Rutgers University by Hildegarde E. Peplau.
1963	Perspectives in Psychiatric Care published; Journal of Psychiatric Nursing and Mental Health Services published.
1973	Standards of Psychiatric–Mental Health Nursing Practice published, certification of psychiatric-mental health nurse generalist established by American Nurses Association.

KEY POINTS

- First institution for the mentally ill was opened in London as **the Bethlehem Royal hospital** in 1247.
- **Philippe Pinel** (1745-1826), a French physician who advocated moral treatment in mental health care.
- **Benzamine Rush** referred to as the "Father of American Psychiatry" wrote the first American text book of psychiatry.
- **Linda Richards** is called the first American Psychiatric Nurse.
- **Harriet Bailey** wrote Nursing Mental Disease, the first psychiatric nursing text book in1920.
- The **first school to prepare nurses** to care mentally ill opened at Mc Lean Hospitals in waverly, Massachusetts, in 1882.
- **Hildegard Peplau** (1909-1999) laid the ground work for interpersonal and interactive processes in nurse patient relationship.
- **Hildegard Peplau** (1959) wrote the history of psychiatric nursing.

10 Mental Health and Psychiatric Nursing: Indian Scenario

MENTAL HEALTH SERVICES IN INDIA

Mental health is an integral part of the total health. Till recently, the importance of mental health in the total health was not adequately emphasized. The scope of mental health was confined to some seriously mentally ill patients admitted to the mental hospitals. Mental health did not find its appropriate place in health planning due to a common misconception that prevalence is low in India as compared to western countries and no effective treatment is available for psychiatric disorders. According to various epidemiological surveys done in last 3-4 decades, the magnitude of major psychiatric disorders in India is around 10-20 per thousand of population. If the figure of neurotic and psychosomatic disorder is to be included, number of patients requiring help at any given time increases to 5-10% of the population.

MAGNITUDE OF MENTAL HEALTH PROBLEMS IN INDIA

- Nearly one percent of the population suffers from major mental illness. That means around 10 million suffer from severe mental disturbance in India.
- Around 2-3% percent suffer from mood disorders (especially depression).
- Anxiety and other disorders are found in 8-10 percent of the population.
- Around 3-5 percent of population suffers from ill-effects of excessive alcohol drinking and drug addiction.
- Nearly fifteen percent of the population suffers from some sort of psychological disturbance.
- Dementia is found in 3-4 percent of the subjects aged over 60.
- In children nearly 3 percent suffer from some sort of mental retardation. 5 percent suffer from emotional and conduct disorder.

It is also estimated that around 15-20 percent of people who seek medical help in various health care centers have mild psychological disturbances. But most of them are not aware of it.

Most of the patients with psychiatric disturbance still remain without help for a long time because of illiteracy, stigma, misconception, fear and faulty attitudes regarding mental illnesses. People in our country still believe that mental illnesses are caused by evil spirits, possession of demons, punishments for the misdeeds of ancestors, black magic, witchcraft, bad stars and sins. Therefore, they seek the help of faith healers, temple treatment, tantrics and magicians. Many of them are not aware that it is an illness. While there are millions of people suffering from various types of mental illnesses, the mental health care facilities available in India are meagre.

Resources to deal with this magnitude of problems are limited in India. The hospital based mental health services are mainly of two types Mental hospitals and Psychiatric units of general hospitals. Advances in pharmacological treatment of psychiatric disorders resulted in lesser need of mental hospitals and opening of psychiatric facilities in general hospitals. The last 2-3 decades have seen the gradual and sustained developments of general hospital units. This has been quite successful in improving the mental health services, and has also helped in destigmatizing the mental illnesses to a larger extent.

MENTAL HEALTH IN INDIA –AT A GLANCE

Problem

- 1% of population suffers from Severe Mental Disorders like Schizophrenia and other psychosis (10-12 million).
- About 10% of population suffers from minor mental disorders like Anxiety, Neurotic disorders etc.(100 million).
- 20-30% of patients in general clinical setting are suffering from an Underlying Psychiatric Disorder.
- Suicide rate in India is about 10 per lac population.
- About 1-2% of total children have some underlying psychiatric problem.
- About 0.5-1.0% of all children have mental retardation.

Resources

- About 25000 beds in 37 mental hospitals and 2000 to 3000 psychiatric beds in general and teaching hospitals.
- First mental hospital was built in Bombay (Mumbai).
- In India with population of one billion, there is one psychiatric bed per 30000 population.
- 3500-4000 qualified psychiatrists, 800-1000 clinical psychologists and 600-800 psychiatric nurses, and 600-800 Psychiatric social workers available to look after these problems.
- One psychiatrist per 3-4 lakh population.

MENTAL HEALTH NURSING IN INDIA

Though psychiatric nursing in the West began to emerge as a profession in the late nineteenth century and by twentieth century it had evolved into a specialty with unique roles and functions, yet in India psychiatry nursing was recognized as a specialty area in nursing only in the later part of twentieth century.

Initially there was no component of psychiatric nursing in the nursing curriculum in India till mid of 20th century. The Health Survey Committee's report in 1946 recommended preparation of nursing personnel in psychiatric nursing also. Based on the committee's recommendation, a one year post certificate course in psychiatric nursing was started in 1956 at the National Institute of Mental Health and Neurosciences (NIMHANS), Bangalore, which was later followed by few more centers.

Later, On recommendations of the Mudaliar committee in 1964 and as per requirement of Nursing council that a nursing course should have a mental health component, in the year 1965 the Indian Nursing Council included psychiatric nursing as a compulsory course in the B.Sc. Nursing programme. In 1965-66, psychiatric nursing component was also added to the General Nursing and Midwifery Course. This significant progress in the psychiatric education for nurses was because of a few historical noteworthy events like:

- Introduction and widespread use of psychotropic drugs in effective management of psychiatric patients.
- Felt need of quality care of psychiatric patients in mental hospitals.
- Integration of mental health services in general health services.

By 1980, psychiatric nursing course was included as an elective subject for the students of diploma in nursing education & administration programme and students of M.Sc. Nursing at a few specific centres. Later in revision of the General Nursing and Midwifery (1986) syllabus, the content of psychiatric nursing was dealt with, in more depth. Students are required to take the theory as well as practical examination.

Training nursing students in various psychiatric set-ups provides opportunities for further development of a specialty area in nursing that concentrates on the care and treatment of the mentally ill. In the last few years psychiatric nursing has become an examination subject, and there are Board and University examinations in psychiatric nursing for both Diploma in Nursing and Degree (B.Sc.) students respectively. Thus, psychiatric nursing has emerged as an essential part of the curriculum of nursing education.

In summarization, it is appropriate to say that the need of psychiatric nursing is not only felt at the undergraduate level but also at the post-graduate level. Specialists in psychiatric nursing are expected to teach and participate in the clinical field and do research work in psychiatric nursing.

KEY POINTS

- People in our country still believe that mental illnesses are caused by evil spirits, possession of demons, punishment for the misdeeds of ancestors, black magic, witchcraft, bad stars and sins.
- 1% of population suffers from Severe Mental Disorders like Schizophrenia and other psychosis (10-12 million).
- About 10% of population suffers from minor mental disorders like Anxiety, Neurotic disorders etc.(100 million).
- In India only 600-800 psychiatric Nurses are available to look after the needs of psychiatric patients.
- One year post certificate course in psychiatric nursing was started in 1956 at the National Institute of Mental Health and Neurosciences (NIMHANS), Bangalore.
- In 1965 the Indian Nursing Council included psychiatric nursing as a compulsory course in the B.Sc. Nursing programme. At the same time psychiatric nursing component was also added to the General Nursing and Midwifery Course.

11 Nursing Process in Mental Health

Nurse-patient relationship is an important landmark in nursing process. The nursing process is an interactive, problem solving process and a systematic and individualized way to achieve the outcome of nursing care. In nursing process the nurse and patient develop in a relationship built on trust and directed towards maximizing the patient's strengths, maintaining integrity and promoting adoptive response to stress.

In dealing with mentally ill patients, the nursing process can present unique challenges. Mental health problems show different symptoms which are vague and elusive and not visible like physical symptoms. Many psychiatric patients are even unable to describe them properly. Ability of patient to participate in problem solving process also may be limited because of their impaired touch with reality.

Vital to this process, is the therapeutic climate of interaction between the patient and members of the mental health team that is in contact with the patient. The nurse can initiate and establish a sense of trust by approaching the patient in an accepting and non-judgmental manner. This trusting relationship is vital to the successful outcome of improved functioning and well being of the patient.

STEPS OF NURSING PROCESS

Nursing process is an organized method of problem solving called the care plan. It is developed from information that is gathered during initial phases.

Nursing process consists of five phases:

1. Nursing assessment.
2. Nursing diagnosis.
3. Expected outcome.
4. Nursing Interventions.
5. Evaluation.

1. Nursing Assessment

A basic nursing assessment usually includes detailed psychiatric history and mental status examination of patient. These include both subjective and objective data.

By asking direct leading questions, the nurse gets subjective information of problems concerning the patient. Successful gathering of data is based on ability of nurse to listen to the patient and ensure him privacy and confidentiality.

The **subjective data** include name and general information about the patient, patient's perception of current stressor, current occupation and work history, difficulties in relationship, any somatic complaints, history of substance use if any, interest or activities previously enjoyed or sexual activities or difficulties.

The **objective information** is observed by the nurse or provided by others in the family of the patient. The objective assessment includes physical examination, complete mental status examination, MMSE etc. It is also important to note that verbal communication and non verbal mannerisms, expressions and emotions, while gathering data of objective assessment. A sample of nursing assessment of psychotic patient is outlined in box.

Nursing Assessment of Psychotic Patient

A Nursing Assessment includes a few basic principles which are as follows:

1. Schizophrenia is a psychotic disorder in which patient is not having awareness about his illness, so because of this illness person may not always be a reliable source of information. So a complete history should be taken from family members or other persons familiar to patient.
2. Schizophrenia is a chronic illness needing long term treatment.
3. Identify the type of disturbance the patient is experiencing.
4. Determine the theme and content of delusional thinking, assess the intensity of disturbance and risk for violence.
5. Assess speech pattern.
6. Assess emotions and affect whether they are appropriate in relation to present situation or lack of interest in the environment.
7. Assess biological patterns of patient like sleep habits, eating habits, personal hygiene (self care activity).
8. Determine any suicidal ideation.
9. Observe for posturing or motor disturbances.

2. Nursing Diagnosis

Making nursing diagnosis from collected data is second step in nursing process. A nurse analyzes all data gathered and compares it to normal functioning. A nursing diagnosis is not a medical diagnosis but an identification of patient's problem based on conclusions.

The most commonly used standard is that of the North American Nursing Diagnosis Association (NANDA). A list of common NANDA's nursing diagnosis is given in the box.

Once applicable nursing diagnosis has been determined, they are to be prioritized according to the severity and immediate urgency of the problem. A nursing diagnosis of suicidal ideation or intent would require the nurse's attention first. Based on Malsow's hierarchy of needs, needs of biological domain must have priority over needs of psychological or social domain.

Possible Nursing Diagnoses in a Psychotic Patient

After detailed and careful assessment a nursing diagnosis can be formulated. A nursing care should be planned to focus on symptomatic relief as well, with careful attention to physical, emotional and social needs imposed by impaired mental functioning. Nursing diagnosis for patients with schizophrenia may include:

- Self care deficit.
- Altered nutrition.
- Altered thought due to delusional thinking.
- Impaired verbal communication.
- Altered perception due to hallucinations, illusions.
- Altered affect.
- Violence (Self directed or directed at others)
- Social isolation.
- Low self esteem related to chronic illness.
- Non-compliance to treatment due to denial of illness.
- Hopelessness due to chronic impairment.
- Sleep disturbance.
- Impairment of judgement and attention.

Nursing diagnoses can be grouped under various headings as per patient's need like:

1. **Biological needs**
2. **Psychological needs**
3. **Social needs**
4. **Recreational needs.**

3. Expected Outcome

This phase of nursing process includes planning a realistic and measurable outcome of problems identified in nursing diagnosis. These outcomes are defined in Immediate Goals (IG) and Long Term Goals (LTG). The Immediate goals addresses the immediate unmet needs of the patient and long term goals addresses the maximal realistic achievement for patient at the time of discharge.

A few examples of immediate goals and long term goals are given below:

Immediate outcomes

- To help the patient communicate his problem effectively.
- Patient remains free from harm to self or others in next 48 hours.
- To decrease patient's anxiety level in next 24 hours.
- To help the patient to develop interest in eating.
- Reduction in symptoms of auditory hallucinations.

Long term outcomes

- To develop effective communication ability.
- To enable the patient to lead a productive life.
- To help the patient to develop meaningful relationships with others.
- To develop the contact with reality.
- To help the patient to learn the importance of treatment.

The anticipated outcomes will depend on the level of functioning demonstrated by the patient. This will depend on the severity of symptoms and the effectiveness of antipsychotic drug therapy or other therapeutic approaches. It is important to remember that the goals and time frame for improvement be realistic.

Expected Outcomes for Schizophrenic Patient

Expected outcomes for the schizophrenic person may include that he or she:

- Develops reality based ways to communicate and meet self needs
- Remains oriented to self and the environment
- Interacts appropriately with others
- Does not injure self or others
- Performs self care and hygiene with minimal prompting
- Demonstrates increased trust of others
- Exhibits increased ability to associate behavior with misperceived environmental stimuli
- Participates in unit activities with appropriate behavior
- Identifies realistic self-expectations and perceptions
- Has reduced incidence of hallucinations
- Cooperates with staff in taking medications.

4. Nursing Interventions

This phase includes actions taken by the nurse to assist patient in achieving the anticipated outcome. Nursing interventions are intended to encourage, maintain, and re-establish a level of mental and physical functioning that promotes the wellbeing of the patient. In planning of action, it is important to consider those levels of functioning that are realistic for that person. A written plan should be made after combined efforts between all members of mental health care team. Nursing interventions mainly focus on mental health care including observing behaviors and symptoms, improving communications, asserting in problem solving with improved over all functioning.

This step of nursing intervention should focus on helping patients to rechannel their energy in a constructive manner and resolve the identified problem. For principle of Nursing intervention see table.

Basic Principles of Nursing Intervention

- Respect each patient as he or she is.
- Accept him or her as such.
- Nursing Intervention should be person specific not the symptom specific. Symptoms are important but not as important as person.
- Make frequent contact with patient and have concern about his needs.
- Have patience, move at the patient's pace and ability.
- Be honest with patient so he can rely on you.
- If a patient is violent, hostile and out of control, ask for help.
- Suggesting, requesting, advising or encouraging work better than commanding.
- Use positive reinforcement (Compliment, Reassurance) to modify his or her maladaptive behavior.

5. Evaluation

This is a continuous and ongoing phase in which nurse evaluates the success of the nursing interventions as per the criteria outlined in the expected outcome. A nurse should review on following points

- Goal has been achieved or not?
- Some progress has been made towards intended outcome or not?
- If a goal has been partially met, then plan should be continued or withdrawn.
- Which need to be assessed again, replanned, implemented and re-evaluated again?

CONCLUSION

The nursing process is scientific, organized, problem solving method of addressing those situations for which nursing can legally intervene. The psychiatrist is responsible for treating the medical or psychiatric disorder. As a member of the mental health team, the nurse is responsible for assessing and communicating information concerning the current status of the patient to the team.

KEY POINTS

- **Nurse-Patient relationship** is an important landmark in nursing process.
- The **nursing process** is an interactive, problem solving process and a systematic and individualized way to achieve the outcome of nursing care.
- Nursing process consists of five phases: **Nursing Assessment, Nursing Diagnosis, Expected Outcome, Nursing Interventions** and **Evaluation.**
- A basic nursing assessment usually includes detailed psychiatric history and mental status examination of patient. These include both subjective and objective data collection.
- For **nursing diagnosis**, a nurse analyzes all data gathered and compares it to normal functioning. A nursing diagnosis is not a medical diagnosis but an identification of patient's problem based on conclusions.
- Nursing diagnoses can include various domains like **Biological, Psychological, Social and Recreational domain.**

- Outcomes in nursing process are defined in terms of Immediate Goals (IG) and Long Term Goals (LTG).
- **Nursing interventions** are intended to encourage, maintain, and re-establish a level of mental and physical functioning that promotes the wellbeing of the patient.
- **Nursing interventions** mainly focus on mental health care including observing behaviors and symptoms, improving communications, assisting in problem solving with improved over all functioning.
- **Evaluation** is a continuous and ongoing phase in which nurse evaluates the success of the nursing interventions as per the criteria outlined in the expected outcome.

12 The Therapeutic Relationship and Communication

The therapeutic relationship is a basic requirement of nursing practice. The therapeutic relationship is seen as a helping relationship in which one person assists in the personal growth and improved well-being of the other. In the nurse- patient relationship, a series of interactions between the nurse and patient provides information about the patient's need and problems. The nurse works in collaboration with other members of the mental health team; towards a common goal of assisting the patient in adaptive and improved functioning.

On the contrary social relationship is a relationship with mutual interests, which satisfy needs of each other and may exist life long.

COMPONENTS OF THE NURSE-PATIENT RELATIONSHIP

Empathy

The establishment of a therapeutic nurse patient relationship is dependent on certain consistent behaviors by the nurse. Among them one of the important is empathy. To hear what another person is saying, to have access to that person's feelings temporarily, and to perceive the situation from that person's perspective is vital to the establishment of trust. At the same time, it is important for the nurse to maintain objectivity and remain in touch with their own feelings. To become sympathetic and mild into the patient's problem is non therapeutic.

Acceptance

Nurse's acceptance of the patient as person with worth and dignity who is not judged and labelled by the nurse's standards is necessary for the establishment of a trusting climate. It is the nurse's willingness to recognize the emotionally ill person as one who deserves respect and needs approval that helps the patient to begin trusting the environment. Foundations of a therapeutic relationship are honesty, integrity, consistency. The patient needs constant reassurance to develop a sense of emotional security within the environment.

Self-Awareness

It is an important aspect of a nurse which she must identify in herself. Self-awareness is a consciousness of a one's own individuality and personality. Knowledge of self as whole person can became a reality only with a gradual awakening to oneself. We cannot have an understanding of others unless we learn about ourselves. Awareness of oneself as a whole person comes with an attitude of openness and wanting to come to an honest evaluation of behavior of self. A desire to make changes in self is also an essential component. We must listen to our daily record of self-talk and be willing to change our recurrent negative scripts. When we move beyond ourselves and see the world from the perspective of others, we open the door for growth. The key is in our thinking. It is the same honesty and openness we try to elicit in our patients who have emotional and mental issues.

Rapport

Rapport, interpersonal harmony characterized by understanding and respect, is important in trusting therapeutic relationship. Nurses establish rapport through interpersonal warmth, nonjudgmental attitude and by showing understanding. Patients with mental disorders often feel alone and isolated. When rapport develops, a patient feels comfortable and secure and finds easy to disclose about himself.

Essential components of a therapeutic relationship

- Empathy
- Caring
- Acceptance (unconditional positive regard)
- Mutual trust
- Honesty
- Integrity
- Consistency
- Genuineness
- Self-awareness
- Limit-setting
- Reassurance
- Explanations

PHASES OF A THERAPEUTIC RELATIONSHIP

Therapeutic relationships are dependent on the situations and needs of the individual patient. The phases of this nurse-patient relationship focus on the patient's ability to function in the process. The therapeutic nurse patient relationship consists of three major and overlapping stages or phases of contact with the patient.

Orientation Phase

This phase involves getting to know the patient. It involves an explanation of the purpose for the nurse patient interactions as means of establishing trust. The nurse and patient contract a time and place for meeting, during which the focus is the patient's problem. The nurse's role is to be a facilitator. Confidentiality is explained in terms of information that is shared only with members of the treatment team as it applies to patient's well-being.

It is important to assess the content of any negative feelings the patient may be experiencing while reinforcing the limits for behavior. These initial data provide a baseline for the next phase of the relationship. It is essential for the nurse to convey a caring and honest concern for the client and sending a congruent message through both verbal and nonverbal communication. By showing a genuine interest and supportive attitude, the nurse helps the patient to feel worthwhile.

Working Phase

This is a stage of identification and exploration of problems. This is a period in which outcomes and interventions toward behavior change are planned and goals are developed to improve the well-being of the patient. This involves work by the nurse and the patient to develop an awareness of the problem and solution to it. Through the use of problem solving skills, the nurse assists the patient to express feelings and thoughts about the present situation. It is important for the nurse to model and teach appropriate coping skills. The patient is encouraged to practice adaptive responses and evaluate the effectiveness of the changes. Every effort should be made to reinforce and support, each small step of the patient. Helping the patient to set priorities, provides a way of accomplishing short term gain towards a bigger step or challenge.

Resolution Phase

The third phase or termination phase of the relationship allows the patient to depend on his or her own strengths, while developing improved adaptive skills. The nurse should encourage the patient to have increased social interactions and participate in all activities.

This promotes independence, getting along with others in preparation for discharge and a return to the demands of society. It is not uncommon for nurses to feel like they are abandoning the patient's trust as a therapeutic closure occurs. The nurse should let the patient know that the relationship was valued and purposeful in helping the patient toward relying on his or her own ability to deal with problems.

PROFESSIONAL BOUNDARIES FOR HELPING

It is essential for the nurse to remember that the needs of the nurse are distinctly different from those of the patient. Some interventions are helpful and promote independence but others actually allow the patient to develop a dependence on the nurse patient relationship. As patients improve, they are expected to function independently. The nurse cannot let the relationship fulfill a personal need and remain objective about the patient's needs at the same time. Anytime the nurse shows more concern for one patient over another, he or she is at risk for becoming too involved. When focus on the patient is maintained, it is less likely that the nurse will be manipulated into violating a professional boundary.

The nurse patient relationship must not extend beyond the therapeutic termination phase. Any further contact by phone, mail, or socialization is in violation of the professional code of ethics. If a former patient is seen outside of the mental health setting, it is import- ant to avoid recognition or speaking to them unless they recognize and speak first. Detailed conversation or other interactions should be avoided.

THERAPEUTIC COMMUNICATION

The nurse patient relationship is built on therapeutic communication. Therapeutic communication is an ongoing process of interaction through which meaning emerges. Effective communication skills include verbal and nonverbal techniques. The principles of therapeutic communication are given in Box.

The principles of therapeutic communication

1. Patient should be primary focus of interaction.
2. A professional attitude sets the tone of therapeutic relationship.
3. Self disclose cautiously and only if it has a therapeutic purpose.
4. Maintain confidentiality.
5. Asses patient's intellectual competence to determine the level of understanding.
6. Avoid social contact with patient.
7. Maintain a nonjudgmental attitude.
8. Guide the patient.

Therapeutic and social relationships are very different. In a therapeutic relationship, nurse focuses on the patient and patient related issues, even when engaging in social activities with that patient.

VERBAL COMMUNICATION

The process of verbal communication includes a sender, a message and a receiver. The patient is often a sender and nurse is often a receiver. The patient's word and their underlying emotional tone communicate the underlying individual's need and emotional problems. The nurse receives the message, decodes it and then responds to the patient. Validation is essential to ensure that the nurse has received the information accurately.

Self Disclosure

One of the most important principles of therapeutic communication for the nurse to follow is to focus the interaction on the patient's concerns. Self disclosure, telling personal information of self to the patient is not a good idea. The conversation should focus on the patient, not the nurse. Nurse sometime may feel uncomfortable avoiding patient's questions for fear of seeming rude. Nurse may need to tell the patient that nurse will not share the personal information.

VERBAL COMMUNICATION TECHNIQUES

Psychiatric nurse uses many verbal techniques in establishing relationship and helping patients focus on their problems. These techniques at first seem artificial, but with practice, they can be useful.

Silence

One of the most difficult but often most effective technique is the use of silence during verbal interactions. By maintaining silence, nurse allows the patient to bring his thoughts together and proceeds at his or her own pace.

Listening

Listening is an ongoing activity by which the nurse attends to the patient's verbal and nonverbal communication. The art of listening is developed through careful attention to the content and meaning of the patient's speech. There are two types of listening–passive listening and active listening. The **passive listening** involves sitting quietly and letting the patient talk. Passive listening does not foster a therapeutic relationship and usually communicates a boredom, indifference, or hostility.

Active listening focuses on what the patient is saying to interpret and respond to the message objectively. While listening, the nurse concentrates only on what the patient says and the underlying meaning. The nurse's verbal and nonverbal behavior indicates active listening. Some verbal techniques block interactions and inhibit therapeutic communication. Such verbal techniques are giving advice to patient, agreement with patient's view point, challenging patient's view point, judging patient's situations etc.

NONVERBAL COMMUNICATION

Gestures, facial expressions, and body language actually communicate more than verbal messages. Under best circumstances, body language mirrors what is verbally communicated. When verbal and nonverbal messages are conflicting, the listener should believe the nonverbal message. People with psychiatric problems often have difficulty in verbally expressing themselves and interpreting the emotions of others, nurse needs to assess continually the nonverbal communication needs of the patients.

Eye contacts, facial expressions, movements, postures and gestures are nonverbal behavior that communicates thoughts and feelings. Patients with low self-esteem may be unable to maintain eye contact and spend a great deal of time looking towards the floor. A patient pacing and restless may be having a reaction to medication. A cultural context of body language should also be taken in to consideration in communication. Nurse should use positive body language. Generally nurse should not cross arms or legs during therapeutic communication, because such postures crect barriers to interaction.

KEY POINTS

- **The therapeutic relationship** is seen as a helping relationship in which one person assists in the personal growth and improved well-being of the other.
- **Essential components of a therapeutic relationship are** empathy, caring. Acceptance (unconditional positive regard). Mutual trust, honesty, integrity, consistency, genuineness, self-awareness, limit-setting, reassurance and explanations.
- **To deal therapeutically with the emotions, feelings and problems of patients, nurse must understand their own cultural values, beliefs, interpersonal strengths and limitations.**
- To be sympathetic and mild into the patient's problem is non therapeutic approach.
- **In a nurse-patient relationship, as in all type of relationships, certain physical, emotional, and social boundaries and limitations need to be observed.**
- The therapeutic nurse patient relationship consist of three major and overlapping stages or phases of contact with the patient:
  1. **The orientation phase.**
  2. **Working phase, and**
  3. **Termination or resolution phase.**
- The nurse patient relationship must not extend beyond the therapeutic termination phase. Any further contact by phone, mail, or socialization is in violation of the professional code of ethics.
- In verbal communication, patient's word and their underlying emotional tone communicate the individual's need and emotional problems. The nurse receives the message, decodes it and then responds to the patient.
- Self disclosure, telling personal information of self to the patient is not a good idea. The conversation should focus on the patient, not the nurse.
- Eye contact, facial expression, movements, postures and gestures are nonverbal behaviors that communicate thoughts and feelings and under best circumstances, body language mirrors what is verbally communicated.
- Nurse should use positive body language. Generally nurse should not cross arms or legs during therapeutic communication, because such postures erect barriers to interaction.

13

Mental Health Team and Role of Nursing

Mental health care is an integration of various approaches that have been developed, to meet the demands of mentally ill patients and their family members. In the past, those with mental illness were kept away from society and locked in institutional settings. Now with better understanding of etiological factors and symptomatology of mental illnesses, the present trend is to recognize the disorders as treatable illnesses with more favourable outcomes.

Patients with need of mental health care have the right to humane and individualized treatment plans. Recent studies have shown that mental illness accounts for more than one-fourth of all cases of disability in United States, Canada and Western Europe. Although treatment may be available, a large percentage of people with mental illness are either not receiving or getting treatment. There continues to be a need to improve public understanding, attitudes, and actions to fight stigma attached with mental health and illness.

The goals of treatment are designed to reduce the symptoms of mental disorders and to allow those who suffer from these disorders to live and function in society with improved personal and interpersonal skills. There are many specific types of therapies that may be used by various mental health professionals of the treatment team.

MENTAL HEALTH TEAM

Within the various mental health care settings such as psychiatric hospitals, private nursing homes, mental health clinics, and social service agencies, helping professionals work together and provide a coordinated approach towards a common outcome of improved access to treatment for those needing care. The members of mental health team are:

Psychiatrist: A psychiatrist is a physician licensed to practice medicine and specializes in psychiatric or mental disorders. A psychiatrist can evaluate, diagnose, and treat all types of mental illness, including pharmacological, biomedical and psychotherapeutic interventions. Some psychiatrists sub-specialize in the pediatric, adolescent or geriatric sector of population. Psychiatrist serves as a leader of mental health team.

Clinical psychologist: Most licensed clinical psychologists have received a master's or doctoral level degree specializing in clinical psychology with advanced training and field requirements. These professionals administer and interpret psychological testing that can be used in the diagnostic process. The clinical psychologist also provides individual, family and group therapy to assist in the resolution of mental health issues.

Psychiatric nurse clinical specialist: Psychiatric nurse clinical specialist should have a masters degree in nursing with post graduate research work. She coordinates community mental health and participates in primary, secondary, tertiary prevention of mental disorders. She also conducts individual, group and family therapy sessions in hospital and community settings.

Psychiatric nurse: Psychiatric nursing is a specialized area of nursing practice, that focuses on the prevention and treatment of mental health related problems. Most psychiatric nurses are registered nurses who have gone through a General nursing and midwifery programme or B. Sc Nursing programme with an elective course in psychiatric nursing. Nurse develops skills in caring for mental patients in mental hospital setting, and helps in various coordinated activities of wards. She also coordinates with clinical nurse specialist in community mental health delivery.

Psychiatric social workers: Clinical social workers usually have a master's or doctoral level degree in psychiatric social work and are trained as patient's advocate. Their role includes assessing the individual, family and community support system, and helping in discharge planning, and counseling of job placement etc. The social worker works with placement agencies, such as community group homes and nursing homes, to secure a continued support and care system for the patient who is unable to live in an independent or home setting.

Occupational therapist: Occupational therapists have a bachelor's or master's level degree in occupational therapy. They have an important role in assessing patient's capabilities and skills in different areas and helping them to develop specific skills in areas of their choice. They work with patients to improve their level of functioning for everyday living. Activities such as cooking, money management, grocery shopping, and transportation are used to improve self-esteem and promote a realistic level of independent living. Occupational therapist works with other members of the team towards rehabilitation and discharge planning.

Dietician: Dietician usually has a master's level degree in nutrition. They serve as a resource person by providing nutrition information and counselling to patients with specific nutritional problems and needs.

The mental health treatment team

- Psychiatrist
- Clinical psychologist
- Psychiatric nurse
- Psychiatric nurse clinical specialist
- Psychiatric social worker
- Vocational nurse
- Mental health technician
- Professional counsellor
- Recreational specialist
- Occupational therapist
- Clergyman
- Dietician.

ROLE OF NURSING IN MENTAL HEALTH CARE

As a member of mental health team, the psychiatric nurse play a variety of different roles. Advances in the past few decades in field of psychiatry and in nursing have reemphasized the role of nursing in various settings. The role of psychiatric nurse is changing from providing services to patients in custodial care to giving care to patients in community. The increased awareness of mental disorders in society and growing demand of quality services for patients has changed the conventional role of nurse.

The nurse patient therapeutic relationship provides multiple opportunities for the nurse to obtain information that is often a vital source to other team members. Information may be communicated verbally or documented in the medical record. This may be helpful for various intervention strategies. The nurse also serves a liaison between the patient and therapist. The nurse assesses, evaluates and interacts with patient on a day-to-day basis. The nurse is a vital component of maintaining a therapeutic environment. In addition the nurse helps the patient in communication skills and social interactions with others in the milieu. In all, nurse promotes a positive outcome for the patient and their family. A brief discussion of various roles of nurse is as follows:

As Caregiver

The nursing process provides the foundation for the implementation of all nursing interventions. Basic to the nursing assessment is the observation of appropriate and inappropriate behaviors, noting both precipitating factors and situational reinforces. This information is documented in the patient record and provides feedback to other members of the mental health care team for evaluating effectiveness and progress of the treatment plan. A response to therapy is often observed by the nurse while performing other nursing interventions such as medication administration, physical assessment, or assisting with personal care. It is important for the nurse to positively reinforce appropriate behavior and encourage patients to participate in all aspects of the psychotherapeutic process.

As Counsellor

Nurses is often the person who is available and willing to provide an attitude of genuine concern for the patient through active listening and therapeutic communication. The patient should be encouraged to openly express feeling and thoughts without reprisal.

As Educator

Nurses are often the link between patients and information about their illness and treatment. Compliance with treatment is more probable when patients are informed about the problem and how the treatment works. Education is provided at the patient's level of understanding through verbal explanation, demonstration and printed materials about the illness and treatment regime. It is important for the nurse to evaluate the patient's understanding of the instructions by verbal response or return demonstration.

As Advocate

As a patient's advocate, the nurse functions to protect the rights of the patient through acceptance and support for decisions that are made. The treatment compliance usually improves as the nurse demonstrates an empathetic positive regard for patient needs. Empathy involves the nurse's willingness to understand the situation from the patient's perspective.

KEY POINTS

- Team approach is significant in mental health care.
- The members of mental health team are Psychiatrist, Clinical Psychologist, Psychiatric Nurse, Psychiatric Nurse, Clinical Specialist, Psychiatric Social Worker, Mental Health Technician, Professional Counselor, Recreational Specialist, Occupational Therapist, Clergyman and Dietician.
- The nurse is a vital part of the mental health care team.
- The nurse plays a daily interactive role with the patient, providing a therapeutic atmosphere in which assessment and evaluation of behaviors and communication skills is facilitated.
- The therapeutic process focuses on interactive relationships between a mental health practitioner and the patient, with an expected outcome of reducing the effects of the emotional disturbance or disorder and improving both the personal and social well-being of the patient.

- Individual psychotherapy focuses on the problems or situations with which the patient is having difficulty: it guides and assist the patient to work towards resolution of the road-blocks in mental functioning.
- Other types of therapy, such as group, family, play, or recreational therapy, and biofeedback, may be used to address contributing issues.
- A combination of these psychotherapeutic methods combined with the benefit of psychotropic drugs provides an effective treatment for the patients with mental health disorders.
- The ultimate goal of all treatment regimes is improvement in personal and social functioning of each patient at optimal and satisfying level and nurse plays a vital role in achieving this goal.

14 Interview Techniques and Psychiatric Assessment

Assessment is the collection and interpretation of biopsychosocial information to determine health, functional status, and human response to mental health problems. Assessment is not an isolated activity. It is a systematic and ongoing process that occurs throughout the nurse's care of the patient. Assessment has many purposes. It may be comprehensive or short and focussed. Assessment begins with the first contact with the patient and may incorporate different methods of data collection.

A thorough psychiatric assessment consists of psychiatric history taking, mental status examination, complete physical examination, and selected laboratory and psychological test screening of the individual. Psychiatric history is of crucial importance as it is the most important tool to arrive at nursing needs, planning of nursing care, interventions and implementation of nursing care plan, and evaluation of care given.

OBJECTIVES OF PSYCHIATRIC EVALUATION

- To make a nursing diagnosis.
- To find out the precipitating factor and primary cause of behavior.
- To estimate the severity of patient's condition.
- To decide on an initial course of action and to plan nursing interventions.
- To develop a relationship with the patient.
- To engage the patient in psychotherapy.

A. HISTORY TAKING

- **Interview Setting**

Psychiatric interview is different from other medical disciplines, because here we wish to obtain information about patient's behavior, his problems against his wishes. A proper setting of interview would facilitate good outcome.

It is important that patient should be made comfortable during the interview. The interview should be conducted in a separate room, where repeated interruptions should not take place because interruptions will disrupt the flow of interview. Always ensure confidentiality except in cases of suicidal /homicidal risk and child abuse. The sitting arrangement could be around the table. It is better to seat the patient on the right side of the table, so that the nurse can restrain the patient, if needed. The table should not have loose objects.

- **Nurse-Patient Relationship**

Interview process involves the following:

a. *Nurse:*
   - Must have training for becoming a skilled interviewer.
   - Training should include learning about her own reactions and prejudices and to develop therapeutically condusive temperamental qualities.
   - Should not evaluate patients on her personal scale.

- Learn to respect her patients, their belief and life style.

b. *Patient:*
- His reaction towards nurse may be positive, negative or ambivalent.
- Few patients expect the nurse to do something, while he remains the passive recipient. The patients come to the mental health care centre with the expectations that all his difficulties will be resolved promptly, which create a false hope.
- Others may be more active and cooperative in treatment.

c. **Informants:** Psychiatric patients are often not in a position to give a detailed account of their problems due to lack of insight or their uncooperative attitude. When a patient is accompanied by relatives, history should be obtained from them also. Reliability of information given should be determined by asking a few questions regarding his education, duration of their stay with patient, his/her relationship with the patient and their concern about the patient. If the accounts of different informants are consistent, then the information may be considered reliable.

IDENTIFICATION DATA

Identification data includes Name, Age, Sex, Marital status, Education, occupation, Income, Residential address, Official address, Type of family, Date of admission and Identification marks.

PRESENTING COMPLAINTS

The patient should be asked for reasons for consultation. Presenting complaints must be recorded in their chronological order of appearance with duration. All complaints must be recorded in patient's own words and use of technical terms should be avoided.

HISTORY OF PRESENT ILLNESS

This section of history taking provides a detail of presenting complaints with duration, variation in severity from day to day and with in a day, aggravating and relieving factors, impact of complaints on patient's social and occupational functioning. A detailed account of treatment received with type and doses of drugs are also recorded in this section.

PAST HISTORY

Details of past history of psychiatric illness, if any, should be recorded in this section with type of treatment and response to it. A detail history of past medical illness if any, needs to be noted.

FAMILY HISTORY

This part of history includes recording of age, status of physical and mental health, education, occupation, income and personality of parents and siblings. The family history of mental illness, alcoholism, epilepsy or other significant illness should also be recorded. Type of family (Nuclear or joint or extended nuclear), environment and socioeconomic status of family are also important part of this section. A family tree can be used to describe the number of family members, their age, history of mental illness and any death occurring in the family.

PERSONAL HISTORY

This section of history helps to understand the patient's complaints in light of patient's personal history. Information should be gathered under the following headings:

Antenatal History

- Condition of mother during pregnancy.
- History of stressful factors during pregnancy.
- Type of delivery-normal or complicated.

- Was the patient a wanted or unwanted child?
- Did child cry just after birth?
- Did he achieve all milestones at appropriate age?
- What was the patient's infantile pattern of activities?

Childhood History

- Relationship of child with his parents and other family members.
- Was patient affectionate, trusting, active, shy, irritable, aggressive or selfish child?
- Were there any neurotic traits like stuttering, enuresis, nightmare, nail biting or thumb sucking?

Schooling History

- Age at entry of schooling.
- Problem in schooling, if any.
- Relationship with teachers or peers.
- Difficulty in academic performance, if any.

Occupational History

- Status of patient at working place.
- Work or job satisfaction.
- History of change in job.
- Relationship with co-workers.

Sexual and Marital History

- When did he develop sexual interests.
- History of masturbation and associated feelings.
- Age of marriage.
- Relationship with spouse, level of satisfaction with spouse.
- Relationship with children.

Menstrual History

- Age of menarche.
- Reaction to menstruation.

PREMORBID PERSONALITY

It is very important to know about patient's personality before the onset of illness. In this section various dimensions of individual's personality like his social and interpersonal relationships, his predominant mood, intellectual and recreational activities, his attitude towards work, energy initiative, habits and fantasy life should be recorded.

Information on these parameters should be gathered from patient as well as reliable informants.

B. MENTAL STATUS EXAMINATION

A mental status examination is a systemic documentation of the quality of mental functioning at the time of interview. It helps both with current diagnosis and treatment planning and serves as a baseline for future references. The examination includes following:

Appearance, Attitude and Behavior

Appearance: Overall impression of patient like attractive, unattractive, posture, clothes, grooming, facial expressions (alert, dazed, perplexed, frightened) eye contact (eye open, avoids eye contact, stares directly towards examiner).

Behavior and motor activities: Slowness of motor movements or excessive motor activity, gestures, abnormal motor movements like tics, mannerism, stereotyped motor activity or waxy flexibility etc.

Attitude towards examiner: Cooperative or uncooperative, interested or disinterested, hostile or defensive, guarded or evasive etc.

Speech

Pressure, tone, volume of speech is increased or decreased, spontaneous speech is present or absent (mutism).

Flow of speech–smooth or hesitant, sudden blockage in speech, circumstantiality, tangentiality, verbigeration, flight of ideas, clang association etc.

Mood and Affect

Mood is a sustained emotional state like depressed, euphoric, elevated, anxious, angry, irritable. Affect is a patient's current emotional state like appropriate or shallow, flat, blunted, inappropriate.

Always assess appropriateness of affect in relation to situation or thought contents.

Thought

Conventionally in MSE, thought is assessed under following headings:

Form of thought: Does the patient's thinking make sense?

Does one thought follow another thought logically?

Does the patient display–circumstantiality (over inclusiveness in his reply), Loosening of association, tangentiality (thoughts are unrelated but the patient seems unaware of this), Perseveration (needless repetition of same thought or phrase in response to different questions), verbigeration, flight of ideas (rapid jumping from one idea to another idea with understandable association), clang association etc.

These abnormalities are most commonly associated with schizophrenia or affective disorder.

Thought contents: Check for presence of various abnormalities e.g. Abnormal preoccupations, Obsessions (Unwanted, repetitive, intrusive thoughts or images or impulse in spite of patient's effort to get rid of it), Delusions (false, firm unshakable belief that are not shared by others).

Perception

Does the patient have illusions (misinterpretation of a real external stimulus), hallucinations (false perception without an external stimulus). Hallucinations may be Auditory, Visual, Olfactory, Tactile, Gustatory. Hallucinations occurring while a person is falling asleep are called hypnogogic hallucination and those occurring as one is awakening from sleep are called hypnopompic hallucination.

Attention and Concentration

Can patient pay attention for short periods of time (Attention) without being distracted by minor stimuli?

Can he attend it for length of time (concentration)?

Test attention by digit recall (speak a series of numbers in a monotone, and ask the patient to repeat them, begin with three and increase by one with each successful trail. The normal maximum response is six numbers repeated).

Test concentration by serial subtractions test (subtracting serial sevens from hundred or serial three from forty or by asking the patient to count backward from twenty).

Orientation

Whether the patient is oriented to Time (by asking time, date, day, month or year), Place (by enquiring present location), Person (by identifying others in surrounding). Time sense is usually the first to be lost .Major disorientation suggests ogranicity.

Memory

Test all three types of memory: Immediate, Recent, Remote.

Immediate by:

1. Digit repetition.
2. Ask patient to remember 3 objects and 3 words and ask for them after 5 minutes.
3. Ask the patient to count—stop him at 27 (wait for 1 minute) –tell him to continue counting—stop at 42 (wait for 3 minutes—then continue counting).

Recent by:
Ask questions about the past 24 hours—How did you travel here? What was on the news last night?
Remote by:
Asking for personal details like date of birth, date of marriage, last four presidents of country etc.

Intelligence

Intelligence can be assessed by the fund of general information that the patient has, keeping in mind the patient's educational and social background. e.g.—How many weeks in a year? Name the last three prime ministers? What is the function of liver?

Abstract Thinking

Abstract thinking is an ability of a person to find hidden meaning of specific example. The common method of assessing is to give a proverb and ask its meaning. Other way is to find out similarities and differences in sets of object like Baseball/Orange, Car/Train, Table/Chair.

Judgment

Judgment is an ability of person to assess and respond to a situation appropriately. Judgment may be Social and Test judgment.

Social judgment is inferred from behavior, which he shows during personal life situations. It can be assessed by asking questions e.g. What should you do if you find a stamped addressed letter? Or What should you do if you lose a book belonging to a library?

Test judgment is assessed by asking questions that what he will do in a particular situation.

Insight

Insight refers to the patient's awareness and understanding of his illness. Whether he recognizes that he is suffering from illness? If yes, then what kind of illness? Does it require treatment?

Insight is divided into following grades: (i) Complete denial of illness (ii) The patient is uncertain whether he is ill or not (iii) The patient accepts his illness but blames it on other external factors (iv) The patient accepts his illness but cannot pinpoint responsible factors (v) The patient accepts his illness and considers this illness is due to psychological factors (Intellectual insight) (vi) The patient is emotionally aware of his inappropriate feelings or thoughts.

C. PSYCHOLOGICAL ASSESSMENTS IN PSYCHIATRY

The information obtained from history, mental status examinations, physical examination and biological investigations are not sufficient to make exact diagnosis. In this context psychological testing is of particular importance in clinical psychiatry.

Psychological testing of patient is ideally conducted by a clinical psychologist. These tests provide a standardized objective measurement of intelligence, cognition, personality psychodynamics, memory etc. For convenience psychological tests can be grouped into following categories:

1. **Projective tests:** These tests are assessments which elicit responses that can be analyzed for psychodynamic and related contents and reveal that how the subject think, feel and perceive relationships and situations. The common projective tests are Rorschach Inkblot Test, the Thematic Apperception Test, the Sentence Completion Test, Draw a Person Test and Observation of Children at play.
2. **Personality tests:** These tests measure diverse aspects of cognition, affect and conation, including interpersonal and attitudinal characteristics. They also assess personality dynamics, to study the effects of brain damage etc. Many of the projective tests such as Rorschach, TAT, Draw a Person, and sentence completion test have been used in assessment of personality. In recent years, self

administered questionnaires have gained importance as methods of personality assessment. Few important questionnaires are The Eyesenck Personality Inventory (EPI), Cattel's 16-Personality Factor Inventory (16 PF), The Minnesota Multiphasic Personality Inventory (MMPI), Millon Clinical Multiaxial Inventory (MCMI).

3. **Intelligence tests:** Intelligence tests throw light on subject's capacities and aptitudes, whether above or below average. In the latter instance these tests indicate the degree of intellectual subnormality or severity of mental retardation. A few common intelligence tests are described below:
   - **The Binet Kamat test:** The Binet Kamat Test is a test of general intelligence. The performance of a child on the items of this test is compared with age-average norms obtained from children of various ages. A child above average intelligence will therefore have a mental age which exceeds his chronological age; a below average child will have a mental age below his chronological age.
   - **The Wechsler adult intelligence scale:** The Wechsler adult intelligence scale is one of the most popular and widely used intelligence tests. It comprises verbal and performance scales; the former is made up of 6 subtests. The verbal subtests are Vocabulary, Information, Comprehension, Arithmetic, Digit span and similarities. The performance subtests are Block Design, Picture Completion, Digit Symbol, Picture Arrangement and Object Assembly. A modified version of WAIS is available for use in children. It is known as the Wechsler Intelligence Scale for Children (WISC).
   - **Raven's Progressive Matrices:** Raven's Progressive Matrices (RPM) is the closest to being culture free. The most commonly used version of the RPM is the Standard Progressive Matrices. The advanced Raven's Matrices is used in very intelligent adults.
4. **Neuropsychological tests:** Deterioration in intellectual functioning occurs as individuals age, in subjects with disorders such as alcoholism and Schizophrenia, and in patients with overt central nervous system pathology ranging from epilepsy to head injury. Such Neuropsychological assessment is generally carried out using a sophisticated battery of tests. Luria-Nebraska battery, Halstead-Reitan Battery, Michigan Neuropsychological Battery and the Shipley Institute of Living Scale. The batteries used in India are the NIMHANS Neuropsychological Battery, Bender Gestalt Test and PGI Memory Test.
5. **Rating scales:** Rating Scales are instruments used to assess the magnitude or severity of a psychological construct or disorder. While Rating scale does not fall directly under the ambit of psychological testing, they are

Table 14.1: Common rating scales in psychiatry

1. **For the assessment of general mental health:**
   - Goldberg general health questionnaire (GHQ)
   - Subjective well-being inventory (SWBI)
2. **For the assessment of anxiety:**
   - Hamilton Anxiety Rating Scale (HARS)
   - Covi anxiety scale
3. **For the assessment of depression:**
   - Hamilton depression rating scale (HDRS)
   - Beck depression inventory (BDI)
4. **For the assessment of mania:**
   - Young's mania rating scale (YMRS)
   - Bech-Rafaelson mania scale (BRMS)
   - Biegel mania rating scale
5. **For the assessment of Schizophrenia:**
   - Brief Psychiatric Rating Scale (BPRS)
   - Scale for Assessment of Positive Symptoms (SAPS)
6. **For overall assessment:**
   - Clinician's global inventory (CGI)
   - Global assessment scale (GAS)

nevertheless important in several situations. Rating Scales are available for a wide range of disorders, and indeed for a wide range of situations within a given disorder. Common Rating Scales in psychiatry are listed in Table 14.1.

KEY POINTS

- Complete psychiatric assessment include History taking, Mental status examination, Physical examination with relevant Lab and psychological tests.
- Psychiatric evaluation helps in making diagnosis, estimate severity and deciding the management.
- Interview should be conducted in comfortable and cordial environment.
- Always ensure confidentiality except in case of suicidal /homicidal risk and child abuse.
- Role of informant in psychiatric history is important. Always assess informant's reliability and his intention before interviewing him.
- Psychiatric history includes history of present illness, past history, Family history, personal history and assessment of premorbid personality.
- MSE includes patient's appearance, his behavior and mood, abnormality in his thought process and perception, and change in patient's higher mental functions.
- Psychological tests can be used for assessment of patient's personality, Intelligence, and his psychopathology indicating some psychiatric illness.
- Rorschach and TAT are commonly used projective tests for personality.
- The Binet Kamat test, Bhatia's battery test and the Wechsler adult intelligence scale are common tests used for assessment of intelligence (I.Q.).
- Routine tests for investigation of psychiatric patients include Hemogram, Blood sugar, X-ray chest, X-ray skull and ECG.
- Serological tests for HIV, CT scan brain, MRI brain and genetic tests for detecting abnormality are commonly used specific routine tests in psychiatry.

15 Legal and Ethical Aspects of Mental Health Nursing

Psychiatric nurse should be sufficiently aware of the legal and ethical issues pertaining to psychiatry. Care of patients with mental disorders involves a certain set of principles and values. The nurse must have knowledge of the laws and ethical governance of mental health care delivery. Similarly, the nurse is also responsible for maintaining standards within the nursing profession itself. Thus the knowledge of these issues not only protects her from unnecessarily involving in the legal issues, but also helps her to protect the rights of mentally ill patients.

LEGAL ISSUES

Law and psychiatry come face to face at various junctions e.g. in crime committed by the mentally ill, validity of a marriage, validity of a contract, admission of mentally ill persons, validity of a will etc. The nurse working in a psychiatric hospital should know the following basic legal aspects of psychiatry:

- Civil responsibility.
- Criminal responsibility.
- Law related to psychiatric disorders.
- Admission and discharge procedures in psychiatric hospitals.

MENTAL DISORDER AND RESPONSIBILITY

Responsibility, in the legal sense means the liability of a person for his acts or omission, and if these are against the law, the liability to be punished for them. The law presumes that every person is mentally sound until proved otherwise.

A. Civil Responsibility

The question of civil responsibility arises in the following conditions:

1. **Management of property and affairs:** A mentally sick person cannot transfer or sell his property to others. On receipt of an application by the relatives of a person, the court may direct an inquiry to find whether a person is of unsound mind and incapable of managing his property and affairs.
2. **Insanity and contract:** A contract is invalid if one of the parties at the time of making it was incapable of understanding what he was doing due to unsoundness of his mind.
3. **Insanity and marriage:** A marriage is considered invalid, if at the time of marriage either party:
   - Is incapable of giving valid consent due to insanity.
   - Though capable of giving valid consent, has been suffering from such kind or degree of mental **disorders** to be unfit for marriage and procreation, or
   - Has been suffering from recurrent attacks of insanity or epilepsy (The Hindu Marriage Act, Act 25 of 1955 and section 5 II, Act 68 of 1976).
4. **Competence of insane to be a witness:** A person of unsound mind is not competent

to give evidence if he cannot understand the necessity of telling the truth due to insanity. An insane person is competent to give evidence during the period of lucid interval.

5. **Consent and insanity:** Consent to certain acts like sexual intercourse or hurt is not valid, if such consent is given by a person who from unsoundness of mind is unable to understand the nature and consequence of that act.
6. **Insanity and testamentary capacity:** Testamentary capacity (Testament–will) is the mental ability of a person to make a valid will. The requirements for a valid will are as follows:
   - A written and properly signed and witnessed document must exist.
   - The testator must be major i.e. >18 years of age and of sound disposing mind at the time of making the will.
   - Force, influence, or dishonest representation of facts should not have been applied by others.

   If a person suffers from mental illness at the time of making his will and if he does not have the mental capacity to understand the consequences of the act, his will becomes invalid.

B. Criminal Responsibility

A person may plead insanity to avoid:

1. Conviction, if the accused was insane when the alleged crime was committed.
2. Trial, when the accused is insane and cannot plead.
3. Capital punishment, when a condemned prisoner later becomes insane.

Almost all the laws pertaining to the responsibility of the insane in criminal cases are guided by the McNaughten rule laid down in the English court after the McNaughten trial in 1843. According to this Rule.

"An accused person is not logically responsible, if it is clearly proved, that at the time of committing the crime, he was suffering from such a defect of reason from abnormality of mind, that he did not know the nature and quality of the act he was doing, or that what he was doing was wrong"

This legal test has also been accepted in India as the law of criminal responsibility and is included in Sec.84 of the Indian Penal Code (IPC) which is as follows: "Nothing is an offence which is done by a person, who at the time of doing it, by reasons of unsoundness of mind, is incapable of knowing the nature of the act, or that what he is doing is either wrong or contrary to the law".

ACTS OF LAW PERTAINING TO THE MENTALLY ILL

1. **Indian Lunacy Act, 1912:** This was the first Act introduced in India which dealt with the mentally ill persons. It contained 8 chapters, which dealt mainly with the admission, treatment and discharge, establishment of asylums and certain rules regarding the mentally ill persons who were referred to as 'lunatics'.

   This act was riddled with many discrepancies and was in many ways inadequate to take care of the problems of the mentally ill.
2. **Mental Health Act, 1987:** This Act replaced the Indian Lunacy Act of 1912. This bill was introduced in the Rajya Sabha (Bill No. XLI) in 1981 and it became an Act in 1987. It consists of ten chapters.

Chapter-1: Definitions

This gives a brief introduction to the act and certain definitions of terms included in the act. The term 'lunatic' was deleted from this act and replaced by 'mentally ill person'.

Chapter-2: Mental Health Authority

This chapter deals with the proposal to establish a central authority "Mental Health Authority" by central or state government to regulate, develop, direct and coordinate the mental health services.

Chapter-3: Psychiatric Hospitals and Psychiatric Nursing Homes

This chapter deals with criterion and facilities required for setting up psychiatric hospitals and psychiatric nursing homes for the admission, treatment and care of mentally ill persons.

Chapter-4: Admission and Detention in Psychiatric Hospitals and Psychiatric Nursing Homes

This chapter deals with the procedures of admission and discharge of mentally ill persons. Admission in psychiatric hospitals can be done under the following circumstances:

A. **Voluntary basis:** A mentally ill person who is a major can request for admission to a psychiatric hospital on a prescribed form to the medical officer in charge of the hospital. In case of a minor his legal guardian can apply for admission in a psychiatric hospital by submitting the application.

B. **Admission under special circumstances:** In case where the patient is violent or not consenting, the medical officer in charge of the hospital, can admit these persons on the request of relatives and friends if their claim is supported by two medical certificates (one from a gazetted medical officer) for a period not exceeding 90 days.

C. **Temporary treatment order:** This is issued by the magistrate of the area on production of wandering and/or dangerous mentally ill person before the magistrate by the police in charge of police station.

Chapter-5: Inspection, Discharge, Leave of Absence and Removal of Mentally Ill Persons

This chapter deals with the provisions for the appointment of a board of visitors containing not less then 5 visitors of whom at least one shall be a medical officer preferably a psychiatrist for timely inspection of psychiatric hospitals and nursing homes.

Discharge: The medical officer incharge of a hospital can discharge any patient except a criminal with the consent of two medical officers of his team. The patient can also apply for leave of absence if he applies on a prescribed form to the medical officer incharge of a psychiatric hospital.

Chapter-6: Judicial Inquisition

The judicial inquisition regarding alleged mentally ill persons possessing property, custody of his person and management of his property are dealt with in this chapter.

Chapter-7: Liability to Meet the Cost of Maintenance of Mentally Ill Persons

The cost of treatment of mentally ill persons will be borne by the state unless provided by any law for the time being in force.

Chapter-8: Protection of Human Rights of Mentally Ill Persons

This a new chapter added in the Act. According to the new Act:

- No mentally ill person shall be subjected during treatment to any indignity (whether physical or mental) or any cruelty.
- No mentally ill person under treatment shall be used for the purpose of research unless such research is of direct benefit to him for purpose of diagnosis or treatment or such persons being a voluntary person has given his consent in writing or the guardians of the minors have given consent in writing.
- No letters or communications sent by or to a mentally ill person under treatment shall be intercepted, detained or destroyed.

Chapter-9

This chapter deals with the penalties associated with the violation of the Mental Health Act.

Chapter-10

This chapter deals with miscellaneous issues like conduct of a medical officer in charge of a psychiatric hospital and others.

ETHICAL ISSUES

Ethics

The term ethics refers to a set of principles or values that provide dignity and respect to the patient. Ethics also provide a guiding philosophy for the nursing profession and protects patients from unreasonable treatment. Nurses have an obligation to be familiar with the rights of the patient and current laws concerning care.

Patients Rights

Every psychiatric patient receiving treatment has certain rights that have been documented in the report of Human Right Commission and Mental Health Act of 1987. This document is usually displayed in a prominent area of the patient service units so that it is available to patients and families. It is a nurse's responsibility to be familiar with these rights and to ensure that they are preserved and protected. Such rights have been specified in chapter -8 of Mental Health Act 1987.

Right to Appropriate Treatment

Although the nurse is not directly responsible for deciding the place and mode of treatment, yet it is an integral part of the nurse's responsibility to ensure that the patient receives appropriate care. All patients are entitled to receive the best available care based on a current and individualized treatment plan. Patients have a right to:

- Know the qualification of the professionals who are treating him.
- Be treated in the least restrictive setting, one that prevents excessive restrain.
- Know about the side effects of treatment and its cost, plan for him.
- Refuse to be part of a drug trail, experimental therapy or treatment methods.
- Understand the effects of prescribed medications along with any potential adverse effects.
- Refuse treatment unless there is a court order for treatment and admission.

Informed Consent

Prior to admission to any mental health care setting, nurse should obtain informed written consent for various available treatments and procedures. In the case of an incompetent or incoherent patient, a family member or legal guardian should be given this information for their consent. At the same time, the patient has the right to refuse any aspect of treatment and may elect not to sign the consent. At the time of admission to a mental health setting, the patient receives an explanation of the hospital policies regarding available services, various procedures and associated risks, visitation, phone usage, physician contact.

Confidentiality

Confidentiality refers to patient's right to prevent written or verbal communications from being disclosed to outside parties without authorization. The record and correspondence should not be made available to relatives or any third party, as this can be misused by anyone for humiliating the patient or his family or for right of property. To facilitate a patient's trust, nurses must assure her patient that all communication is confidential and will not be communicated to anyone not participating in his care. Every member of the treatment team has a duty to uphold this ethical standard. Protecting the patient's record from unauthorized personnel is a nursing responsibility. Situations that require disclosure of patient information may include:

- When patient is intends to commit a crime.
- When his duty involves the life of a number of persons.
- Infected by life threatening contagious diseases like HIV.
- Evidence of child abuse.

Accountability

Nurses are accountable for the care they provide. Each level of nursing is responsible for adhering to the standard of care that is acceptable for that particular level. The nurse practice guidelines in many countries identify the scope and minimum standards of practice for all nurses. Nurses may be held accountable and liable to any patient for an act of incompetence or negligence in the deliverance of care. In mental health care, nurse is also responsible for knowing institutional and governmental procedures regarding patient admission and rights. If uncertainty exists, the nurse is responsible for securing the correct information from other sources such as other health care professionals, textbooks or manuals.

Admissions and Discharge

A patient has the right to receive treatment in the least restrictive environment that would promote safety and therapeutic care. The type of facility and level of care provided depends on several factors. Psychiatrist makes the determination whether the patient will need to receive inpatient or outpatient treatment. Residential facilities are also available for patients who need to reside in a therapeutic environment for extended periods of time.

Many patients with mental health problems request admission to a psychiatric centre for treatment. A voluntary admission occurs when the patient is admitted based on his or her chosen willingness to comply with the treatment program. In this situation, the physician writes the order for admission and the patient signs and agrees to the term of treatment. The person is then allowed to sign the appropriate documents and leave when treatment is complete. An involuntary commitment occurs when a person is admitted to a psychiatric unit against his or her will. The amount of the time a person can be detained is determined by law.

For an involuntary admission to occur, an evaluation statement that clearly indicates that the person's mental state is a danger to self or others is necessary. The patient can be detained on an emergency status against his or her will. At the end of stipulated period, the patient must either be discharged, given voluntary admission status, or receive a court order to determine if there is a need for continued involuntary treatment.

The procedures of admission and discharge of mentally ill persons in psychiatric hospitals can be seen in Chapters 4 and 5 of Mental Health Act 1987.

Seclusion and Restraints

Sometimes use of seclusion and restraints becomes necessary to treat a psychiatric emergency. Physical restraint refers to the use of mechanical devices to provide limited movement by the patient. Physical restraints are used to prevent harm to self or others and require careful monitoring. These may consist of padded leather or cloth devices for the wrist, ankles, waist, or fingers. Chemical restraint refers to use of medication to calm a patient and prevent the need for physical restrains. Chemical restraint is less restrictive and is generally the initial choice unless the situation warrants otherwise. Restraints are applied only with a physician's order and under the supervision of a registered nurse. These methods are only used when verbal interventions or less restrictive methods of treatment have failed or are not available. Many times the environmental situation or other patients have provoked the behavior. In this case, removing the patient to another area of the unit may allow the patient to regain control without further intervention. The patient is usually given sedating medication to provide a calming effect and assist in behavior control. Continuous monitoring of the patient in restraints or seclusion is mandatory. These methods are discontinued at any time they are seen as ineffective. Nurses should be familiar with the legal implications involved in the use of seclusion and restraint. Patients who are confined without justification or who are subject to inappropriate use of seclusion or restrain can be viewed in a civil court as having been falsely imprisoned. The restraint of patient with inappropriate use of force can be viewed as assault and battery. Having an awareness of how, when, and why to use confining methods will help the nurse avoid litigation for these circumstances.

KEY POINTS

- Indian Lunacy Act was passed in 1912 (16th March) and was applicable to whole of India except Jammu and Kashmir till Mental Health Act came in existence.
- Reception Order means an order made by a Magistrate under the provision of Act for admission and detention of a mentally ill person in a psychiatric hospital or psychiatric nursing home.
- Mental Health Act was passed in 1987 (22nd May). It contains 10 chapters; the term lunatic and asylum used in Indian Lunacy Act (1912) have been replaced by the terms mentally ill persons and psychiatric hospitals.
- Almost all the laws pertaining to the criminal responsibility of the insane in criminal cases, are guided by the McNaughten rule.
- Criminal responsibility of a mentally ill person is covered under section 84 of IPC, which says that "Nothing is an offence which is done by a person who at the time of doing it by reason of unsoundness of mind was incapable of knowing the nature of the act or that what he was doing, was either wrong or contrary to the law". An amendment in 1957 has included irresistible impulses under this section.
- Divorce can be obtained on the ground of incurable unsoundness of mind for a specific continuous period or on the ground of fraud (that one party has hidden the fact of unsoundness of mind from spouse).
- A person of unsound mind is not competent to give evidence if he cannot understand the necessity of telling the truth due to insanity. An insane person is competent to give evidence during the period of lucid interval.
- Knowledge of legal and ethical issues not only protects nurse from unnecessarily involving in the legal issues, but also help her to protect the patient's right.
- Ethics provide a guiding philosophy for the nursing profession and protects patients from unreasonable treatment.

- Prior to admission to any mental health care setting, nurse should obtain informed consent for various available treatments and procedures. In the case of an incompetent or incoherent patient, a family member or legal guardian should be given this information for his consent.
- Confidentiality refers to patient's right to prevent written or verbal communication from being disclosed to outside parties without authorization.
- Situations that require disclosure of patient information (breach of confidentiality) may include:
  - When patient intendes to commit a crime.
  - When his duty involves life of a number of persons.
  - Infected by life threatening contagious disease like HIV.
  - Evidence of child abuse.
- Nurses are accountable for the nursing care they provide, which means they must take responsibility for what they do.
- According to Mental Health Act, 1987, the procedures of admission and discharge of mentally ill persons in psychiatric hospitals can be done under the following circumstances—Voluntary Basis, Admission under special circumstance, and Temporary Treatment Order (Reception order).
- Sometimes use of seclusion and restraints become necessary for patients to prevent harm to self or others or when careful monitoring is required.

16

Organic Mental Disorders

It is a psychological or behavioral abnormality associated with presence of demonstrable etiology in form of cerebral disease, brain injury or other insults leading to cerebral dysfunction. These Dysfunctions may be:

- **Primary** (Due to disease, injury or insult of brain).
- **Secondary** (Behavioral disorders secondary to systemic disease).

PRIMARY DISORDER

In which the disturbance of cognitive function, such as memory, intellect, learning or consciousness are major abnormalities. Examples are: Delirium, Dementia, and Organic amnesic syndrome.

SECONDARY DISORDER

In which main manifestations are in areas of perception (hallucination), thought content (delusion), emotion and/or overall pattern of personality and behavior. The disturbances in cognitive functions are minimal. Examples are: Organic Hallucinations, Organic Delusional Disorder, Organic Mood Disorder, Organic Anxiety Disorder and Organic Personality Disorder.

DEMENTIA

It is a chronic progressive disease of brain with usually irreversible outcome. Dementia is characterized by global impairment of higher mental functions (memory, thinking, orientation, comprehension, learning, language and judgment) without affecting consciousness. It is primarily a problem of old age, seen in 5% of persons above 65 years and 20% of persons above 80 years of age. This disorder is uncommon before the age of 60 years. In recent years this illness is becoming a major problem. The major causes are:

- 65% due to Alzheimer's.
- 15% due to Multi-infarct dementia.
- Rest due to other causes (See list of causes).

CLINICAL FEATURES

- Progressive deterioration of intellectual function (insidious onset).
- Loss of memory–forgets day, telephone numbers, personal belongings, names, occupations, place and work.
- Disorientation to time, place.
- Impaired new learning.
- Person becomes socially disinhibited and impulsive.
- Later on unable to take care of self, and becomes sleepless, restless, and starts wandering.
- Mood—depressed or labile.

TYPE OF DEMENTIA

1. Dementia of Alzheimer's Type (DAT)

It is the most common cause of dementia responsible for more than 50% cases of dementia. This disease is also popularly known as "The

Table 16.1: Causes of dementia

1. Neuro–Degenerative disorder • Alzheimer's disease • Parkinson's disease • Pick's disease • Huntington's disease • Progressive supranuclear palsy • Amyotrophic lateral sclerosis • Leuko dystrophy • Wilson's disease • Lewy body disease
2. Vascular dementias • Multi–infarct dementia • Lacunar infarct dementia • Binswanger's Disease • Cortical micro infarction
3. Infections • HIV disease • Creutzfeldt—Jacob disease • Viral encephalitis • Chronic meningitis • Neurosyphilis
4. Drugs and toxins • Alcohol • Analgesics • Bromide intoxication • Benzodiazepines • Carbon monoxide • Psychotropic drugs
5. Intracranial • Tumors • Brain abscess • Subdural hematoma
6. Normal pressure hydrocephalus
7. Nutritional disorder • Wernicke–Korsakoff syndrome • B_{12} deficiency • Pellagra
8. Metabolic and endocrinal disorder • Chronic hepatic encephalopathy • Dialysis dementia- severe renal insufficiency • Wilson's disease • Thyroid and parathyroid dysfunction • Cushing's disease
9. Chronic Inflammatory Disorders • Multiple sclerosis • Whipple's disease.

disease of Century". The exact prevalence of this disease is not known in India. The features include multiple cognitive deficits including memory impairment. The average life span after the diagnosis of Alzheimer's disease is 7-10 years.

Causes

A. **Genetic factor:** Genetics play an important role in this type of dementia. About 40% of patients have family history of DAT. The studies show that Amyloid precursor Protein (APP) gene is related to causation of Alzheimer's disease.

B. **Neuropathological factor:** Alzheimer is characterized by diffuse cortical atrophy. The sulci are flattened and cerebral ventricles are enlarged. The microscopic features are presence of senile (amyloid) plagues, neurofibrillary tangles and granulovacuolar degenerations, which are pathognomic features of Alzheimer's disease.

C. **Neurotransmitters:** It has been observed that Acetylcholine is hypoactive in this disease.

Clinical Picture

Memory disturbance is the most salient feature of this disorder. It is also one of the earliest symptoms. It starts as forgetfulness that gradually increases to the extent that person loses memory for personal details and data. The orientation to time, place and person is also affected. As disease advances patients also display personality changes like becoming moody, introverted, disinhibited, irritable and explosive. Many patients have hallucinations and delusions. Patient may also have aphasia, apraxia and agnosia.

Till date DAT is not a treatable disorder. However number of drugs (Donepezil, Galantamine, Rivastigmine, Tacrine) are being used for this disease, but proven efficacy of these agents is yet to be established.

2. Dementia in HIV Disease

A disorder characterized by cognitive deficits meeting the clinical diagnostic criteria for dementia and also has established diagnosis of HIV infection.

HIV dementia typically presents with forgetfulness, slowness, poor concentration and difficulty in problem solving and reading. A typical affective disorder, psychosis or seizure may be presenting features in few HIV infected subjects. HIV dementia generally progresses quickly to severe global dementia, mutism and death.

3. Multi-infarct Dementia

The multi-infarct dementia is a form of vascular dementia, where the onset of dementia is gradual and often there is history of several episodes of brain ischemia of minor nature. MID constitutes 10-15% of dementias. These multiple infarction leads to progressive stepwise disruption of brain function (step ladder pattern). The detail clinical history, CT scan brain and EEG helps in diagnosis. The management includes treatment of underlying cause.

DIFFERENTIAL DIAGNOSIS

1. Normal ageing.
2. Pseudo dementia.
3. Delirium.

Management

- Find out the cause (after history and investigations).
- If cause is treatable, then start specific treatment as prescribed by the physician.
- Pharmacotherapy:
  - For sleep
  - For behavioral problems
  - For depression.
- Nursing care
  - Good nutrition
  - Family support
  - Family counselling.
- Care in old age home.

Table 16.2: Difference between dementia and pseudo dementia

	Dementia	*Pseudo dementia*
Onset	Gradual, slow progression of symptoms	Sudden, rapid progression of symptoms
Presentation of symptoms	Tries to conceal symptoms	Patient complains much of cognitive loss
Past history	No past history of depression	Past history of depression is present
Appearance and behavior	Neglected and apathetic	Sad, worried look
Response to questions	Angry	I don't know response
Intellectual performance	Global impairment	Complaints are confined to memory

Table 16.3: Difference between dementia and delirium

	Dementia	*Delirium*
Onset	Insidious	Acute
Duration	> 1 month	< 1 month
Orientation	Mostly intact	Impaired
Thinking	Organized	Disorganized
Attention	Intact	Poor
Awareness	Intact	Fluctuating
Perception	Hallucination not present	Hallucinations usually present
Sleep wake cycle	Usually normal	Always disrupted

NURSING MANAGEMENT OF DEMENTIA

The effectivity and safety are main concerns of nursing management for the care and support of patients with dementia and their families. The nursing process includes:

1. Assessment

Nursing assessment of patient with dementia includes a complete present and past history with present mental status examination. Family members are to be included in obtaining history concerning recent memory loss. Nurse should also identify the primary care-giver, support system and knowledge base of the family members. The role of caregiver to the demented patient is a difficult, stressful and time consuming task. A spouse or adult children often assume this role. It is important for the nurse to actively listen to the feeling and concern of the family members and help them. Other important areas to be assessed are impairment in consciousness, mood changes, fear and frustration level, inability to concentrate, agitation, self-care deficit, inappropriate social behavior pattern, judgment ability, sleep disturbances, speech and language impairment, hallucinations, bowel and bladder incontinence, recognition of family members, and any decline in nutritional status etc.

2. Nursing Diagnosis

The frequently changing needs of these patients present a challenge for nurses in all settings. Every patient must be viewed from the perspective of his or her own particular situation. The common nursing diagnoses in different domains include:

Biological Domain

- Imbalance nutrition (Less or more than body requirement).
- Self-care deficit (bathing / grooming /Toileting etc.).
- Bowel/bladder dysfunctions.
- Disturbed sleep pattern.
- Impaired physical mobility, pain and chronic pain.
- Ineffective health maintenance.

Psychological Domain

- Impaired memory.
- Disturbed thought process.
- Chronic confusion.
- Disturbed sensory perception.
- Risk for violence (Self-directs or directed to others).
- Ineffective sexuality pattern.
- Ineffective individual coping pattern.
- Hopelessness.

Social Domain

- Impaired social interaction.
- Social Isolation.
- Risk for loneliness.
- Ineffective coping.
- Hopelessness.
- Powerlessness.

3. Expected Outcomes

Immediate outcome for the patients may include:

- Decreases anxiety level.
- Remains safe and free from injury.
- Does not harm self and others.
- Maintains participation in self care activities.
- Remains oriented to surroundings.
- Follows scheduled routine activities.
- Feels valued and accepted.

A final outcome is that the caregiver and family will identify and utilize community support systems.

4. Nursing Intervention

A. **Interventions for safe environment and healthy communication:**

One of the most important aspects of caring for the person with dementia is communication. Both verbal and nonverbal approaches must be adopted during nursing interventions.

- Use supportive, nonhurried, relaxed body language with a pleasant affect.
- Introduce yourself and call the person by name at each meeting.
- Speak clearly, softly, and, slowly using short simple words and sentences.
- Avoid questions that challenge memory.
- Use face-to-face contact.
- Keep clocks, pictures, calendars in view to help the patient identify with reality and remain oriented with surroundings.
- Play soft music, which has a soothing effect, or the television can be turned on without sound. Misleading stimuli such as excess noise can produce agitation.
- When the patient is delusional, acknowledge his or her feelings and reinforce reality or divert attention to another issue.
- Recognize the patient's feelings and redirect attention to another subject that is pleasant if a patient becomes verbally aggressive.

B. **Interventions for self care:** As dementia advances, the ability to carry out self-care independently is diminished. Nursing interventions that may support the patient's self-care deficit include:
   - Allow patient time to perform those tasks he or she is able to do.
   - Help the patient to brush his teeth and take bath.
   - Assist with dressing-minimize the choices by selecting items of clothing. Different color items help the patient to separate socks from pants. Avoid tight clothing or complicated zippers.
   - Use a same-sex person to give a bath to the patient, which is sometimes accepted better by the patient.
   - Use tub baths, because many patients with dementia are frightened by the falling water of a shower on their skin.
   - Allow rest periods between activities-fatigue produces negative behaviors.
   - Use a bed closer to the floor to prevent serious injury when ataxia is present.
   - If patient's activities are restricted, give massage at the back and frequently change the posture to prevent bedsores.
   - In winter provide adequate clothing, because patient may not ask for it.
   - As dementia progresses, the ability to locate the bathroom and follow through with the steps of toileting is lost. Nurse can best assist the demented patient by doing the following:
     – Label the bathroom door with a picture or large print wording.
     – Assist with clothing fasteners-simplify clothing (e.g., using pants with an elastic waist).
     – Watch the patient for nonverbal message such as fidgeting with pants, increased pacing, going in and out of doors.

C. **Interventions for nutritional care:** Nursing interventions related to maintaining adequate nutritional intake may include:
   - Ask for patient's likes and dislikes.
   - Provide soft and frequent meals.
   - Face the person if feeding, a side approach may frighten the patient.
   - Prevent the patient from eating nonfood items such as napkins, food wrappers, or plants.
   - Consider a mechanical alteration in food consistency as the disease progresses, because swallowing may be impaired.

DELIRIUM

Delirium is the most common organic mental disorder of acute onset, which is characterized by disturbances of consciousness, attention, perception, thinking, memory, emotion and sleep wake cycle. It is a common condition in medical and surgical inpatients wards, where 5-10% of inpatients develop varying degrees of delirium. It is usually a transient condition with complete recovery in 4 weeks.

The important causes of dementia are given below:

Causes of Delirium

1. **Intracranial causes:** Epilepsy, brain trauma, meningitis, encephalitis, neoplasm, vascular disease like-stroke, cerebral abscess or neoplasm.
2. **Drugs and toxins:** Alcohol, anticholinergics, anticonvulsant, antihypertensive, antiparkinsomnias, antipsychotic drugs, steroid, tricyclic antidepressant.
3. **Endocrinal dysfunctions:** Like hypo or hyperactivity of thyroids, parathyroids and pituitary abnormality.
4. **Metabolic causes:** Electrolyte Imbalance and Metabolic Disturbance due to any causes.
5. **Nutritional deficiencies:** Thiamine deficiency, Nicotine acid deficiency, B_{12} deficiency.
6. **Systemic infections:** Acute or chronic septicemia, acute severe systemic infections etc.

Clinical Features

A cognitive disorder with relatively global impairment, consisting of deficit of attention (poor attention and concentraiton), arousal, consciousness, memory (impairment in recent recall), orientation (disorientation to time, place and person), perception (visual hallucination) and speech or language. Changes in sleep wakefulness cycles and abnormal psychomotor activities are also frequent. Onset is typically rapid and course is rapidly fluctuating ordinarily the condition is reversible.

Course

- Mostly reversible.
- In some cases may progress to dementia.
- Sometimes followed by depression or PTSD.
- 10-30% progress to coma or death.

Management

Management of delirium include following measures:

- Identification of cause and their correction.
- Good nursing care (good nutrition, maintenance of fluid, electrolyte are essential).
- Kept in dimly light room in night.
- Frequent reassurances and explanations from staff are helpful.
- To control agitation and insomnia, use Haloperidol (Oral/ parentral) or Diazepam (Oral/IV) under guidance of treating doctor.

OTHER OMD

1. **Organic amnesic disorder:** The important characteristic of this syndrome is impairment of short term and recent past memory with clear consciousness. The important causes are Thiamine deficiency as in chronic alcoholism, brain trauma, cerebral neoplasm, cardiovascular disease, brain hypoxia, multiple sclerosis etc. Management includes treatment of underlying cause e.g. use of Thiamine 100mg/day in Wernicke-korsakoff syndrome.
2. **Organic delusional disorder:** It is characterized by persistent or recurrent delusions without major disturbance of consciousness, orientation and memory (Resemble Schizophrenia). The causes may be Hallucinogens, amphetamine, cannabis, alcohol and temporal lobe lesions. Management includes treatment of underlying cause and symptomatic relief with antipsychotics.
3. **Organic hallucinations:** It is characterized by recurrent hallucinations of any sensory

modality (usually visual or auditory) due to underlying organic cause without major disturbance of consciousness, orientation and memory or mood. The causes include Alcohol, LSD, Cocaine, Cannabis, Phencyclidine, Brain tumors of occipital region, Sensory deprivation and Epilepsy.

Management includes treatment of underlying cause and symptomatic relief with Antipsychotics.

4. **Organic mood disorder:** It is characterized by prominent and persistent mood disturbances without major disturbance of consciousness, orientation and memory (Resemble Affective disorder). The mood disturbance can be depression or mania. The etiological causes are drugs (all drugs known to cause depression or mania), tumors, Endocrinal disorders, infections, vitamin deficiencies and central nervous system disorders.
5. **Organic personality disorder** and **organic anxiety disorder** are other organic mental disorders which resemble functional personality disorders and anxiety disorders. The causes are some identifiable organic factor. Management includes treatment of underlying cause and symptomatic relief with Antianxiety and Antipsychotics.

NURSING MANAGEMENT OF DELIRIUM

Nursing Assessment

In nursing assessment of delirium at first it is important to determine the cause of disorientation and cognitive decline. Nurse plays an important role in obtaining information and assessing patient. Assessments include a complete history and physical examination. If patient is unable to provide adequate information, other family members may be enquired.

Nursing Diagnosis

Each situation of delirium differs from the other, but there are some commonalities in patients of acute confusion. Nursing diagnosis of delirious patient may include:

Biological Domain

- Acute confusion.
- Disturbed sleep pattern.
- Disturbed thought process.
- Disturbed sensory perception (visual or auditory).

Psychological Domain

- Ineffective coping.
- Disturbed personality identity.

Social Domain

- Interrupted family process.
- Ineffective protection.
- Risk of injury.

Expected Outcome

Once problems are identified, the planning for realistic outcomes can be done. Initial and long-term outcome for the patient may include:

- Remain safe, secure from harm or injury.
- Proper orientation of time, place, person and situation.
- Adequate sleep.
- Respond appropriately to incoming stimuli.
- Identify the fear.
- Maintain ideal body weight.

Nursing Interventions

Most of the patients with delirium require specific care to ensure that the permanent damage is avoided. Because the course of delirium is short and critical, the nursing intervention should be immediate and directed towards correction of underlying cause. Specific intervention for delirious patient may include the following:

- Regular monitoring of level of consciousness.
- Provide adequate lighting in patient's room with minimal environmental noise.
- Provide regular verbal, visual or tactile stimulation with frequent interaction with the patient.
- Give regular reorientation of time, place and date by providing calendar, clock and other items.
- Provide glasses and hearing aids to facilitate orientation.
- Ensure safety measures.
- Maintain fluid and electrolyte balance, adequate nutrition and measures to prevent aspiration.

Evaluation

Effectiveness of nursing plan can be assessed by successful reversal of underlying problem. Most of the patients with delirium have a full recovery except in elderly people.

KEY POINTS

- Organic Mental Disorders (OMD) are psychological or behavioral abnormalities associated with identifiable transient or permanent dysfunction of brain.
- Common Organic Mental Disorders are Delirium and Dementia.
- Celsus coined the term 'Delirium' and 'Dementia'.
- Delirium is the most common type of organic mental Disorder.
- Delirium is a disorder of acute onset and characterized by clouding of consciousness, disorientation to time, place and person, distractibility and is associated with perceptual disturbances like illusions and hallucinations.
- 10-15% of all patients in medical and surgical inpatient wards are estimated to develop delirium.
- The major areas of concern in nursing care of patients with delirium includes safety, altered thought process, perceptual alterations, self care deficit, and nutritional problems.
- Effectiveness of care plan can be evaluated by degree to which successful reversal of underlying problems is achieved.
- Dementia is a chronic organic mental disorder of insidious onset characterized by impairment of intellectual functions, impairment of memory, deterioration of personality and lack of personal care. Such patient does not show impairment of consciousness.
- Alzheimer's disease is the most common cause of presenile and senile dementia accounting up to 50-60 % of all causes. The most characteristic feature of Alzheimer's are senile plaques, neurofibrillary tangles and granulovaculor degenerations.
- Multi Infarct Dementia (MID) is the second most common cause of dementia accounting for 10-15% of all cases. This is typically characterized by an abrupt onset, acute exacerbations, stepwise deterioration (Step Ladder Pattern) of clinical picture.
- The most common cause of organic amnesic disorder is thiamine deficiency due to alcoholism.
- Normal pressure hydrocephalus, hypothyroid dementia, toxic dementia are common reversible and treatable dementias.
- It is the responsibility of the nurse to initiate interventions, to whatever degree possible, improve the quality of patient's life and that of family.

17 Schizophrenia

DEFINITION

Schizophrenia is a major psychiatric disorder with varied presentations, which primarily affects thought, perception, affect, mood, behavior and reality testing. Term Schizophrenia means "Schiz – Split" and "Phren –Mind" as splitting of mind functions.

HISTORY OF SCHIZOPHRENIA

History of schizophrenia is as old as history of psychiatry itself. The magnitude of this disorder consistently attracted the attention of major figures in history of psychiatry. **Benedict A. Morel (1809-1873)**, a Belgian Psychiatrist, first used the term "demence precoce" for chronic deteriorating patients whose illness had begun in adolescence. Karl Kahlbaum (1828-1899) described the symptoms of catatonia; and Ewold Hecker wrote about extremely bizarre behavior of hebephrenia. **Emil Kraeplin**, a German in 1896 further differentiated the major psychiatric disorder into two clinical types: (i) Dementia Precox and (ii) Manic Depressive Psychosis. **Eugen Bleuler** first coined the term Schizophrenia and replaced the term "Dementia Precox" in literature. To explain further history Bleuler described specific primary symptoms of schizophrenia in form of Four As. Beside this he also described accessory symptoms of schizophrenia (Table 17.1).

Table 17.1: Bleuler's primary (fundamental) and secondary (accessory) symptoms

Primary symptoms – 4A's
- Associational Disturbances (Particularly loosening of association)
- Affective disturbances
- Autism
- Ambivalence

Secondary symptoms
- Hallucinations
- Delusions
- Negativism.

Kurt Schneider described a number of First Rank Symptoms (FRS) that he considered in no way specific for schizophrenia but of pragmatic value in making diagnosis (Table 17.2). Schizophrenia, Schneider pointed out, can also be diagnosed exclusively on the basis of second rank symptoms and on otherwise typical clinical appearance.

EPIDEMIOLOGY

Prevalence

Schizophrenia is prevalent in all cultures and religions and prevalence rate is similar in all countries. Lifetime prevalence of schizophrenia is about 0.5 to 1 percent. Pooled studies show an incidence of approximately 1 per 1000 population.

Age and Sex

Schizophrenia is equally prevalent in men and women. Men have an earlier onset of schizo-

Table 17.2: Schneider's diagnostic criteria for schizophrenia

Kurt schneider criteria

1. First Rank Symptoms (FRS)
   - Audible Thoughts
   - Voices arguing or discussing or both
   - Voices commenting
   - Somatic passivity experiences
   - Thought withdrawal and other experiences of influenced thought
   - Thought broadcasting
   - Delusional perceptions
   - All other experiences involving volition, made affects, and made impulses
2. Second Rank Symptoms (SRS)
   - Other disorders of perception
   - Sudden delusional ideas
   - Perplexity
   - Depressive and euphoric mood changes
   - Feeling of emotional impoverishment
   - "…. And several others as well"

phrenia than do women. The peak ages of onset for men are 15 to 25; for women are 25 to 35. The onset of schizophrenia before age 10 or after age 50 is extremely rare. Migration, Industrialization and Urbanization have often been implicated to be associated with increased risk of developing schizophrenia. The illness carries a better prognosis in rural societies and developing countries.

Seasonality of Birth

Persons who later have schizophrenia are more likely to have been born in the winter and early spring and less likely to have been born in late spring and summer.

Socioeconomic Considerations

It has been observed that a disproportionate number of schizophrenic patients are in the lower socioeconomic classes. This observation has been explained by the "Downward drift hypothesis" suggesting that affected individual either moves into lower socioeconomic class or fails to rise out of lower socioeconomic class.

Etiology

The cause of schizophrenia is currently unknown. However the fast paced developments in neurosciences combined with advances in psychiatric research have resulted in discovering the causes. In this section, the main etiological theories of schizophrenia are examined.

A. **Biological**

- Genetics.
- Viral hypothesis.
- Immune dysfunction.
- Neuro anatomical theories.
- Neuro chemical theories.
- Neuro developmental.

1. **Genetics:** A wide range of genetic studies strongly suggested a genetic component to the inheritance of schizophrenia. The prevalence of schizophrenia in genetically linked specific population is as follows (Table 17.3).

Table 17.3: Prevalence of schizophrenia

Population	*Prevalence*
I. General population	1%
II. Non twin siblings of a schizophrenic patient	8%
III. Child with either schizophrenic parent	14%
IV. Dy-zygotic twin of schizophrenic patient	12%
V. Child of both schizophrenic parents	40%
VI. Monozygotic twin of a schizophrenic patient	47%

2. **Neuro anatomical (Brain imaging):** The studies using Computed Tomography (CT), Magnetic Resonance Imaging (MRI), in schizophrenic populations have shown the most convincing data that brain of schizophrenic patients have lateral and third ventricular enlargement and some degree of reduction in cortical volume. Many researches using Positron Emission Tomography (PET) to study schizophrenia have measured either glucose utilization

or cerebral blood flow and the positive finding included hypo activity of frontal lobes, impaired activation of certain brain area and hyperactivity of basal ganglia relative to the cerebral cortex.

3. **Neuro chemical:** Number of neurotransmitters have received the attention in schizophrenia research. Among all "Dopamine Hypothesis" is most studied and convincing. This hypothesis posits that schizophrenia results from Dopaminergic over activity at post synaptic receptors. Recently serotonin has become of much interest in schizophrenia research, since the observation that many of the atypical antipsychotics have potent serotonin related activities. Other Neurotransmitters studies for possible etiological role in schizophrenia are acetylcholine, Norepinephrine, GABA etc.
4. **Viral hypothesis:** The suggestion that psychotic illness may be related to an infectious process has a long history. In early part of century, Karl Menninger observed an association between onset of schizophrenia and influenza epidemics. In addition it has also been known that clinical features of viral encephalitis may include psychosis and other features resembling those of schizophrenia.
5. **Immune dysfunction:** Several research groups are exploring the possibility that schizophrenia may be associated with impaired immune function including alterations in autoimmunity. Anticardiolipin antibody and antinuclear antibody, two antibodies that are used as markers of autoimmune vulnerability, have been shown to be increased in patients with schizophrenia in a few studies.

B. **Psychosocial:** According to psychoanalytic theory, a crucial defect in schizophrenia is a disturbance in ego organization, which affects the interpretation of reality and the control of inner drives. Freud believed that schizophrenic patients regress to a phase of primary narcissism and ego disintegration. The concept of ego disintegration refers to a return to the time when the ego was not yet established. The person is unable to develop a mature ego capable of interpreting reality.

According to learning theorists, children who later have schizophrenia learn irrational reactions and ways of thinking by imitating parents who may have their own significant problems. The poor interpersonal relationship of schizophrenic person is also because of their poor role models in early childhood.

CLINICAL FEATURES

The clinical signs and symptoms of schizophrenia raise three important issues:

- No clinical sign or symptom is specific for schizophrenia.
- Patient's symptoms change with time (variability of symptoms).
- Clinician must take into account the patient's educational level, intellectual ability and cultural background.

Normally schizophrenia is characterized by disturbance occurring in several areas of psychological functioning. These areas are as follows:

- Disturbance in general appearance and behavior.
- Disturbance of language and communication (Dis. Form of thinking).
- Disturbance in content of thought.
- Disturbance in perception.
- Disturbance in affect.
- Disturbance in volition.
- Disturbance in motor behavior.
- Disturbance in cognition.
- Other features.

Disorder of General Appearance

Overt behavior of patients may appear normal so that a casual observer may consider them normal, although closer observation for reasonable period is essential to detect abnormality in behavior. Many patients may appear unconcerned with the surrounding. They may be unkempt or untidy with large beard, dirty look in appearance. A few patients may show marked over activity, excessive talkativeness, abusiveness and destructiveness. A small percentage of patients may exhibit symptoms of catatonia (detail in disturbances of volition).

Disturbance of Language and Communication (Form of Thinking)

Some patient may not be speaking (mute) at all or speaking in monosyllables, whereas others speak excessively. Disorder of thinking is the corner stone of the schizophrenic illness. These disorders are mainly inferred from speech or other activities. Common disturbances of thought process are:

- **Irrelevant speech:** The patient does not answer questions appropriately. The speech is not easily understandable. For instance, if the examiner asks the patient to tell his name he may reply "The moon is going down into the river. All men are worthless."
- **Incoherent speech:** The answer of the patient starts relevantly but the later sentences do not have any relation with each other.
- **Loosening of association:** This means that the normal association process is disturbed and this leads to irrelevance, or incoherence or both.
- **Circumstantiality:** The disturbance is characterized by the inclusion of unnecessary details in the answer although the answer is relevant to the question to a great extent.
- **Tangentiality:** The patient's answer may just touch the point but later, deviate to related, but not required details.
- **Neologism:** Some patients develop a morbid habit of coining new words by condensing two or more words, which may not appear meaningful to others.
- **Verbigeration:** The patient repeats one or two meaningful phrases repetitively.
- **Word salad:** Incomprehensible mixture of words.
- **Poverty of thought:** These patients present with impoverishment of thoughts and as such they are found to be frequently repeating one or two ideas or sentences.
- **Thought block:** The patient may stop abruptly while talking and after a few seconds, he may be able to complete the answer. On being asked why he stopped, the patient will say that all of a sudden his mind went blank.
- **Perseveration:** The phenomenon is characterized by patient's repetition of the answer to a previous question. For instance the examiner asks the patient to tell his name and he tells his name but later on being asked where he lives, he may again repeat his name.
- **Poor abstraction:** Abstraction is the ability to identify commonness as well as differences in various things, object or concepts. The schizophrenic often lack this ability. To asses it, the patient may be asked to tell the similarities between orange and banana (both are fruits), bird and airplane (both can fly) or difference between chair and table. Similarly they may not be able to give abstract meaning of simple common proverbs.
- **Thought being read:** The patients complain that other people mysteriously come to know, whatsoever they are thinking, without the former disclosing the same. Some may complain that their thoughts are broadcast on Radio or Television.
- **Thought withdrawal:** Some patients complain that the their thoughts are withdrawn or stolen by some external agency.

Disturbance of Thought Content

- **Delusions** are false, firm unshakable belief of morbid origin which is out of keeping with patient social and cultural background. The delusions can be varied in schizophrenia-persecutory, grandiose, religious or somatic.
- **Delusion of control:** Patient has false feeling that one's will, thoughts, or feelings are being controlled by external forces. The thought withdrawal, thought insertion and thought broadcasting are type of control seen in patients.
- **Ideas of reference:** Patient may think that other people, the television, or the newspapers are making reference to him.

Disturbance of Perception

- It is another commonly observed phenomenon during which the patient experiences perception without a stimulus (hallucination). This disorder of perception or hallucination can occur in any sensory modality e.g. hearing (auditory), seeing (visual), smelling (olfactory), and taste (gustatory) or touch (tactile). In case of schizophrenia, hallucinations are usually auditory (e.g. voices accusing, threatening or commenting on the patient's behavior). Typical hallucinations seen in schizophrenia are "Running commentary on patient's behavior", these voices will repeat what the patient is doing or thinking; they may also advise or direct the patient. Two voices may discuss about the patient and comment on him. The patient may complain that the hallucinating voices are coming from his chest or stomach.

  Visual hallucinations are rare. Though there can be hallucination in other modalities, if hallucination of touch and smell are present, it should strongly suspect an organic illness.

Disturbance in Affect

Most patients of schizophrenia have flattening of affect. These patients appear emotionally indifferent to most of the situations or circumstances. Some may, however, show affect of extreme fear, or perplexity or depression. These affective states are usually not appropriate to their thoughts and often the patient is unable to explain as to what is making him fearful, anxious or depressed. There could be silly, purposeless laughter or giggling in some case.

Disturbances of Volition

- Disturbances in goal directed, self initiated activity or lack of will often contribute to impairment in work performance and causes deterioration of functioning in various roles.
- It can take the form of inadequate interest or drive (avolition) and inability to complete the activity once initiated.
- Other specific kinds of disturbances in volition, like automatic obedience is seen in catatonic schizophrenia.

Disturbances in Motor Behavior

- Motor activities can be decreased dramatically (as in catatonic stupor) or increased as in excitement during the acute stage of the illness.
- Mannerisms, grimacing and stereotypes are characteristically seen in hebephrenic or disorganized schizophrenia.
- Certain other specific motor disturbances like waxy flexibility and posturing are seen in the catatonic subtype.

Disturbances in Cognition

- Schizophrenic patients often have impairments of selective attention and lack of ability to sustain attention and concentration.

- Executive function disturbances are also seen and the ability to change strategies in response to alternation in task is often affected.
- Chronic patients tend to have more cognitive impairments than those in acute phase of the illness.

TYPES OF SCHIZOPHRENIA

Depending on predominant clinical features seen on history and mental status examinations, following subtypes of Schizophrenia are recognized.

Paranoid Schizophrenia (F 20.0)

- Common type of Schizophrenia.
- Onset in late twenties.
- Prominent delusions of persecution or grandiose type.
- Auditory Hallucinations (Voice commanding or threatening).
- Affect is usually hostile or suspicious.
- Prognosis is better than other type of schizophrenia.

Disorganized (or Hebephrenic) Schizophrenia (F 20.1)

- This type of schizophrenia has an early onset, often in early adolescence.
- Rapid progression of symptoms and deterioration of personality.
- The patients are usually incoherent and irrelevant and show poverty of speech.
- Thought disturbances are prominent.
- Mannerism and grimaces are common.
- Emotional disturbances are in form of self absorbed constant smiling and frequent giggling.
- Severe deterioration in activities of daily living like bathing, dressing, grooming etc.
- The illness has a continuous course without any remission.

Catatonic Schizophrenia (F 20.2)

- Type of schizophrenia becoming uncommon gradually. It is characterized by psychomotor disturbances.
- Psychomotor disturbances are in form of catatonic excitement (over activity) or catatonic stupor (hypo activity).
- Catatonic features include mutism (verbally unresponsive), rigidity (heightened motor tone), posturing (maintaining odd posture), grimacing (odd understandable facial expression), echolalia (imitates the examiner's speech), echopraxia (imitates the examiner's action), stereotypy (repetitive, non-goal directive motor activity), Mannerism (odd, purposeful movements), passive active negativism (passive or active resistance to instruction), waxy flexibility (patient maintains the uncomfortable posture for prolong period) and automatic obedience.

Residual or Chronic Schizophrenia (F 20.3)

- Characterized by affective flattening, psychomotor under activity, lack of initiative, poverty of speech, poor eye-to-eye contact and decline in self care and social performance.
- Negative symptoms such as flat affect, alogia, apathy, amotivation and avolition, eccentric behavior as well as social withdrawal are predominant.

Simple Schizophrenia (F 20.6)

- A rare type of schizophrenia.
- Absence of florid symptoms like delusions and hallucinations.
- Characterized by insidious decline in work and overall functioning (Social and occupational).
- Shallowness of emotional responses, indifferences to social responsibilities, absence of will and drive are prominent.

Positive and Negative Schizophrenia

Crow divided schizophrenia syndromes into two types as positive and negative:

Positive schizophrenia: It is characterized by positive symptoms like hallucinations, delusions, and gross thought disorders and respond well to treatment and have better outcome.

Negative schizophrenia: It is characterized by negative symptoms like affective flattening, poverty of speech, lack of initiative, withdrawn and avoidance of social contact and human relationship. These patients tend to show enlarged lateral verticals on CT Scan and respond poorly to treatment.

Undifferentiated Schizophrenia (F 20.3): General features of Schizophrenia are present but may not show symptoms of any of the above subcategories are included in this group.

COURSE AND OUTCOME

Schizophrenia is generally considered to be a chronic illness. It starts with episodic course and later becomes persistent and chronic. Initially it was thought that all schizophrenics show a chronic deteriorating course, but a number of outcome studies indicate a better outcome of schizophrenia these days. About one third of patients recover well, one third continue to experience symptoms but remain functioning and rest one third have a deteriorating course and show disabilities in rest of life. The following factors influence the outcome of schizophrenia in a better way.

Good prognostic factors of schizophrenia

1. Acute onset
2. Presence of precipitating factor
3. Late age of onset
4. Absence of family history
5. Prominent affective symptoms
6. Absence of negative symptoms
7. History of good premorbid (Social and occupational) personality
8. Good social and family environment
9. Good drug compliance
10. Regular occupational history.

OTHER PSYCHOTIC DISORDERS

Every psychotic disorder is not Schizophrenia or Mania. There are a number of psychotic disorders, which do not fulfill the diagnostic criteria of schizophrenia and mood disorder, but exhibit psychotic symptoms. The important psychotic symptoms are:

- Loss of contact with reality.
- Gross disturbances in social, interpersonal and occupational functioning.
- Features like delusion, Hallucination or mood disturbances etc.
- Impaired judgment.
- Unawareness of change in behavior (loss of insight).

Numbers of conditions having these symptoms are as follows:

1. **Schizotypal disorder:** A rare condition in which person exhibits the odd behavior and thinking, somewhat similar to those in schizophrenia but not having characteristic features of schizophrenia.
2. **Persistent delusional disorder:** This is a condition in which individual presents with a persistent single delusion or a set of related delusions. Here persistent means a delusion must be present for at least 3 months. In general a delusional disorder begins in middle or late adult life and overall frequency in male and female is the same.
3. **Acute and transient psychotic disorders:** According to ICD-10 a class of patients developed acute psychotic disorder having acute onset and associated identifiable acute stress. This class does not show features specific of schizophrenia and affective disorders and usually have a better outcome than schizophrenia.
4. **Induced delusional disorder (Folie A Deux):** A rare delusional disorder where the delusions are shared by two or more persons. Only one of the pair suffers from a genuine psychotic disorder, but the other one who has

a dependent relationship with this person starts showing the same. The recommended treatment approach is to separate the affected individual from the source of the delusions and the dominant person should be treated appropriately.

5. **Schizo-affective disorder:** The term "Schizo-affective Psychosis" was coined by Kasanin in 1933. These disorders exhibit symptoms of schizophrenia and mood disorders in the same episodes of illness. The symptoms of both disorders may be simultaneously present or may follow within interval of a few days. It is of three types:
   - Schizoaffective disorder, manic type.
   - Schizoaffective disorder, depressive type.
   - Schizoaffective disorder, mixed type.
6. **Postpartum psychosis:** It is a psychotic disorder seen in women after childbirth and is characterized by confusion, perplexity, mood lability, delusions, hallucinations and depressive features and sleep disturbances. The prevalence of this disorder is 1-2 per 1000 deliveries.

MANAGEMENT OF SCHIZOPHRENIA

The management of Schizophrenia can be divided into three phases:

1. Effective control of acute symptoms.
2. Maintenance phase.
3. Relapse prevention.

   1. **Control of symptoms**

   Treatment setting: As soon as patient comes for treatment or is brought by family members for treatment, the clinician has to decide whether the patient has to be treated as outpatient or to be hospitalized. If patient is excited, violent harmful for self and family, having intention to suicide/homicide then patient should be hospitalized and in condition where patient gets good support of family, his drug compliance can be assured, and he can be safeguarded against harming himself or others then patient has to be treated as outpatient.

   Pharmacotherapy: A wide range of antipsychotics are available for effective control of symptoms in schizophrenia. The newer antipsychotics (atypical) are preferred over the conventional antipsychotics (typical) because of better side effect profile. Among conventional or typical antipsychotic low potency agents are more sedating and have high anticholinergic activities (i.e. chlorpromazine, thioridazine etc.), while high potency agents cause more Extra pyramidal symptoms and tardive dyskinesia (i.e. Haloperidol). The newer atypical antipsychotics that are in common use are Risperidone, Olanzapine, Quetiapine, Ziprasidone and Clozapine. Clozapine is used for class of patients who had not shown beneficial effect on conventional antipsychotics. Clozapine therapy needs a regular monitoring of blood counts because of its effect of agranulocytosis. The list of few commonly used antipsychotics with doses is shown in table:

Antipsychotic drugs	*Common side effect*
Atypical Antipsychotics	
1. Olanzapine	Wt. gain, sedation
2. Risperidone	Wt. gain, sedation
3. Quetiapine	Mild wt. gain, sedation
4. Ziprasidone	Sedation, EPS
5. Clozapine	Wt. gain/ sialorrhea/sedation/agranulocytosis
Typical Antipsychotics	
1. Chlorpromazine	Anticholinergic S.E.
2. Thioridazine	Anticholinergic S.E.
3. Haloperidol	Extra pyramidal S.E.
4. Trifluoperazine	Extra pyramidal S.E.
5. Pimozide	Extra pyramidal S.E.
6. Flupenthixol	Extra pyramidal S.E.
7. Loxapine	Extra pyramidal S.E.

When patient in acute phase of illness presents with excitement, aggression, active delusions and sleep disturbances, antipsychotic drugs should be started immediately.

Mechanism of action: The mechanism for therapeutic action of antipsychotic medications is thought to be as D2 receptor antagonism, preventing the binding of endogenous dopamine to this subtype of dopaminergic receptor. The mesolimbic and possibly the mesocortical dopaminergic, pathways are likely to be the site of action for the antipsychotic effects. Most of neurological and endocrinological adverse effects of antipsychotics can also be explained by blockage of dopamine receptors.

2. **Maintenance phase:** Maintain effective control of symptoms, it is advisable to continue treatment for 6 months to one year for the first episode of illness. If patient has subsequent episodes, it may have to be continued for two to three years. In case of frequent relapses patients may require life long medication.

Treatment of poor compliance patients: Patients who are not compliant with oral medications regularly, need long acting depot preparations. The commonly used preparations are:

- Fluphenazine deconate–25-50 mg I.M once in week.
- Flupenthixol deconate–20-40 mg once in two week.
- Haloperidol deconate–100-200 mg once in a month.
- Zuclopenthixol seconate–200-400 mg in two to four weeks.

Use of anticholinergics: Parkinsonian symptoms can be treated or prevented by adding anticholinergics like trihexyphenydyl (Pacitane), procyclidine (Kemadrine, Dine) or orphenadrine (Disipal). These drugs will generally reduce such symptoms. The use of these drugs is rationalized, when patient is taking high potency conventional antipsychotic drugs like haloperidol, which causes extra pyramidal symptoms.

Role of Electroconvulsive Therapy (ECT): ECT was once used as a major treatment method for schizophrenia, but now has been indicated in following situations:

- Catatonic excitement or stupor not responding to drugs.
- Acutely excited patient not responding to drugs.

3. **Relapse prevention:** The prevention of relapse (re-emergence of psychotic symptoms) is a major challenge in the treatment of schizophrenia. About one fourth of schizophrenics experience exacerbation of psychotic symptoms during one year period even on medications. Psychosocial management plays a crucial role in relapse prevention.

Family Education and Therapy

It is method of educating patient and his family regarding the nature of illness and its outcome. They must be told that this illness tends to have relapses and patient needs a regular supervision and caring attitude. Apart from Psycho education, family members are also be provided social skills training to enhance communication and reduce tension in families. The family with high expressed emotions (EE) (families which display excessive anxiety, over concern, hostility, critical comment and/or over protectiveness towards the patient) has been shown to significantly increase the risk of relapse. Attempts are to be made to decrease the expressed emotions (EE) to protect patient against relapse.

Individual Psychotherapy

In this type of supportive therapy a patient may be involved in man to man relationship with the doctor. The aim of therapy is to help the patient to understand the various difficulties he experiences in his day to day life and to help him to understand misinterpretations. Psychoanalytic psychotherapy is not indicated in management of schizophrenia.

Rehabilitation

Schizophrenia produces long lasting changes in patient's behavior and handicaps him in a number of areas. The social skill training, vocational training and occupational training can help him to rehabilitate. If family support is lacking then patient can be placed in an after care home.

NURSING MANAGEMENT OF SCHIZOPHRENIA

When establishing a nurse-patient relationship with a patient of schizophrenia, it is important to first gain his confidence with your reassuring approach.

Nursing Assessment

A nursing assessment of schizophrenia includes information regarding previous incidence of mental illness or psychotic episode. Looking at nature of illness, patient may not be a reliable informant, family members or other persons familiar to the patient should be consulted. First identify the current problems, patient is experiencing. It is also important to determine the theme and content of thought disorders and assess the nature of threat or risk of violence, if any.

Similarly also assess emotional tone and affect of the patient and their appropriateness to the situation with sleep pattern and interaction with others. Patient's appearance, hygiene and ability to perform self-care should also be assessed.

Assessment of any suicidal intent or recent attempt, if any is also important in case of schizophrenia.

Nursing Diagnosis

After careful nursing assessment and review of information available, nursing diagnosis can be formulated. Nursing care should be planned to focus on symptomatic relief with careful attention to physical, emotional and social need. Nursing diagnosis for patients of schizophrenia in different domains include:

Biological Domain

- Self-care deficit, related to withdrawal or apathy.
- Violence self-directed or directed to others, related to suspiciousness or hallucinations.
- Disturbed sleep pattern.
- Imbalance nutrition.

Psychological Domain

- Altered thought processes related to delusional thinking.
- Disturbed sensory perception for hallucinations.
- Hopelessness.
- Low self-esteem.

Social Domain

- Impaired social interaction.
- Impaired verbal communication, related to fragmented delusional thinking.
- Family process alteration.
- Non-compliance related to denial of illness.

Expected Outcome

Expected outcome will depend on the level of functioning demonstrated by patient, severity of symptoms and effectiveness of antipsychotic drug therapy and other therapeutic approaches. It is important that the goals and time-frame of expected outcome must be realistic. Such outcomes could be immediate and long term outcome.

Immediate Outcome

- Remain oriented to self and environment.
- Interact appropriately with others.
- Has not injured self or others.
- Perform self care and hygiene.
- Identifies realistic self-expectation and perception.
- Has reduced incidence of hallucination.
- Cooperate with staff in taking medication.

Long Term Outcome

- Develop reality based ways of communication.
- Family members to express realistic expectation.
- Perform self care and hygiene.
- Demonstrate increase trust of others.
- Participate in group activities with appropriate behaviour.
- Learn the importance of treatment.

Nursing Interventions

While selecting appropriate interventions for patients, a careful planning is necessary. It is important to avoid over expectations; but at the same time patient should be encouraged to maximize his ability.

Interventions for schizophrenic patients may include:

- Show acceptance of patient, separate the person from his/her behavior.
- Maintain reality based approach to communicate to the patient and talk about his problems.
- Interact with patient on one to one basis.
- Provide a safe environment by removing unsafe objects.
- Provide a non-stimulating environment that reduces external stimuli.
- Acknowledge the perceptional or thought alteration as being real to the patient while reinforcing reality, which helps the patient to recognize symptoms as part of the illness.
- Reinforce the importance of consistent compliance of medications.
- Give the drugs as prescribed by psychiatrist and record and report side effects of drugs.
- Provide positive feedback for appropriate behaviors.
- Encourage the patient to ventilate feelings associated with altered thought and behavior.
- Provide pre-packed food for patients of paranoid schizophrenia, if possible.
- Monitor sleeping hours of patient.
- Encourage participation in social interaction with others.
- Encourage them to maintain hygiene and self-care needs independently.
- Promote patient and family education about illness.
- Monitor patient's fluid intake when patient is violent or in withdrawn state.
- It is important to assess the patient for escalating behavior and intervene before an out of control situation. In some instances patient may be temporarily restrained with.

Evaluation

While evaluating the effectiveness of nursing intervention, nurse should look for the signs of improved functioning of patient. Following signs indicate an achievement of goals set for patients:

- Patient participates in his treatment.
- Appropriate and healthy communication with nurse and other patients is indicative of improved thinking process.
- Any decrease in abnormal behavior indicates a improvement in thought and perceptual abnormalities.

- Reduced suspiciousness is evident by increase willingness to trust staff and other ward patients.
- Better compliance of taking medicines and increase food intake are also indicative of reduced suspiciousness.
- Expression of hopelessness and worthlessness is a positive step as they move towards identification of peer and social support system.
- Involvement in hospital ward activities is a demonstration of their willingness to be engaged in the company of others.

KEY POINTS

- Term 'Schizophrenia' was coined by Eugene Bleuler meaning split- mind.
- The term dementia praecox was coined by Emil Kraepelin.
- Bleuler's classical 4 'As' of schizophrenia are Autism, Affect, Ambivalence and Association disturbances (loosening of association).
- Increased dopamine level is most important biochemical hypothesis in etiology of schizophrenia.
- Catatonic Schizophrenia may present as catatonic stupor (mutism, posturing, negativism, rigidity, waxy flexibility, echolalia) or catatonic excitement (Agitation, restlessness, aggressiveness, pressure of speech and incoherence).
- Paranoid Schizophrenia shows minimum personality deterioration in contrast to other types.
- In Schizophrenia auditory hallucinations are most common types of hallucinations.
- Most frequent symptoms in schizophrenia are lack of insight followed by auditory hallucinations and delusions, but most diagnostic is auditory hallucinations.
- Paranoid schizophrenia is most common and simple schizophrenia is least common type of schizophrenia.
- About one third of schizophrenics recover well, one third continue to experience symptoms but remain functioning and rest one third have a deteriorating course and show disabilities during rest of life.
- Acute onset, presence of precipitating factor, late age of onset, absence of family history, prominent affective symptoms, absence of negative symptoms with history of good premorbid functioning, good social and family environment and good drug compliance are good prognostic factors in outcome of schizophrenia.
- The newer atypical antipsychotics that are in common use are risperidone, olanzapine, quitiapin, ziprasidone and clozapine.
- ECT is indicated in—Catatonic excitement or stupor not responding to drugs and acutely excited patient not responding to drugs.
- The mechanism for therapeutic action of antipsychotic medications is its efficacy as D2 receptor antagonist, preventing the binding of endogenous dopamine to this subtype of dopaminergic receptor.
- Nursing interventions primarily address promotion of self care activities, nutritional correction, proper sleep pattern, protection of patient and others, reality orientation, better communication and social interaction.
- Development of nurse patient relationship becomes key in helping patients manage the disturbed thought and sensory perception.
- Patient and family education are critical interventions for the persons with schizophrenia.

18

Mood (Affective) Disorders

Ordinarily people experience a wide range of moods and have an equally large repertoire of Affective Expression. Let us first distinguish the term 'Mood' from 'Affect'. Mood has been defined as a pervasive sustained feeling tone or emotion, which colors the psychic life of any individual. Affect is the emotional expression associated with an idea.

Affect is a momentary phenomenon whereas mood looks for duration of time. Mood is what is expressed by the individual whereas affect is what is observed by others.

So according to these definitions Depression, Mania, Bipolar Affective Disorders are all examples of mood disorders rather than affective disorders as these were previously known as. Similar changes have been made in new edition of the classification system i.e. DSM IV and ICD-10.

HISTORY

Mood disorders have been existing right from the ancient times. In about 450 B.C., Hippocrates used the term Mania and Melancholia to describe mental disturbances.

The term manic depressive psychosis was first used by Emil Kraeplin.

EPIDEMIOLOGY

The lifetime prevalence of mood disorder has been variously reported as 2 to 25 percent. The lifetime prevalence for major depressive disorders is about 10-25% for women and 5-12% for men. For bipolar affective disorder the lifetime prevalence varies from 0.4% to 1.6%.

CLASSIFICATION

According to ICD-10 Mood (Affective) Disorders are classified as

F 30 Manic Episodes: Includes hypomania, mania without psychotic symptoms, mania with mood congruent or mood incongruent psychotic symptoms etc.

F 31 Bipolar affective disorder: Bipolar affective disorder with current episode hypo manic, manic, mixed or of mild, moderate or severe depression.

F 32 depressive episodes: Depressive episodes of mild, moderate or severe intensity with or without psychotic symptoms.

F 33 Recurrent Depressive Disorders.

F 34 Persistent Mood Disorder: Persistent mood (affective) disorders including Cyclothymia and Dysthymia.

F 38 Other Mood (Affective): Other mood (affective) disorders including mixed affective episodes and recurrent brief depressive disorder.

F 39 Unspecified Mood (Affective) Disorder.

ETIOLOGY

As of now, the exact cause of mood disorder is not known. Over the years a lot of research has been done in trying to find out the etiology of mood disorder resulting in certain theories which will be briefly mentioned here:

Biological Theories

These theories attribute the cause of mood disorder to the dysregulation of various neurotransmitters, alteration of neuroendocrine regulation; sleep architecture disturbances, disturbance in circadian rhythm and to certain neuroanatomical abnormalities.

A. **Dysregulation of neurotransmitters:** Most of the data available are consistent with the hypothesis that mood disorders are associated with dysregulation of neurotransmitters like norepinephrine, serotonin and dopamine. Further inconclusive evidence is available pointing the role of amino acid neurotransmitters like GABA and endogenous opioids in the pathophysiology of mood disorders.
Current hypothesis points that there is depletion of serotonin in the presynaptic neurons in depression, hence the role of serotonin specific reuptake inhibitors in depression which increase the amount of serotonin in the synaptic cleft making more serotonin available to act in the neurons.
As regards dopamine, the data suggests that dopamine activity may be reduced in depression and increased in mania in the mesolimbic region.

B. **Alteration of neuroendocrine regulation:** The major neuroendocrine axes of interaction in mood disorders are adrenal, thyroid and growth hormone axes.
   1. **Adrenal axes:** A correlation between the hypersecretion of cortisol and depression is one of the oldest observations in biological psychiatry.
   Many researchers have noted that a significant proportion (not less than 50 %) of the depressed patients fails to have the normal cortical suppression response to a single dose of dexamethasone (A synthetic analogue of cortisol). This forms the basis of dexamethasone suppression test which was initially through to be of diagnostic utility but is used now as a measure of chances of relapse in a patient with depression.
   2. **Thyroid axis:** Thyroid disorders are often associated with affective symptoms pointing to a relationship between a dysfunctional thyroid axis and mood disorders. About one third of all patients with major depressive disorders who have an otherwise normal thyroid axis have been found to have a blunted release of TSH in response to an infusion of thyrotropin releasing hormone.
   3. **Growth hormone:** Studies have found that depressed patients have a blunted response to noradrenergic stimulation with clonidine induced increase in growth hormone secretion.

Sleep Abnormalities

Many patients with mood disorders have certain characteristic abnormalities in their sleep EEG's. Common abnormalities are delayed sleep onset, shortened rapid eye movement (REM) latency (the time between falling asleep and first REM period); an increased length of the first REM period, and abnormal delta sleep.

Circadian Rhythm

The abnormalities of sleep architecture in depression and the transient clinical improvement associated with sleep deprivation have led to theories that depression reflects an abnormal regulation of Circadian rhythms.

Neuroanatomical Considerations

Biologic research findings support the hypothesis that mood disorders involve pathology of the limbic system, the basal ganglia and the hypothalamus.

Genetic Factors

Genetic data strongly indicate that a significant genetic factor is involved in the development of mood disorder. Family studies indicate that first degree relatives of Bipolar disorder are 8 to 18 times more likely to develop Bipolar disorder and 2 to 10 times more likely to have major depressive disorder than controls.

If one parent has Bipolar disorder, there is a 25% chance that any child has a mood disorder; if both parents have Bipolar disorder there is a 50 to 75% chance that their child has a mood disorder. Twin studies have shown that the concordance rate for bipolar disorder in monozygotic twins is 33 to 90%. For major depressive disorder, the concordance rate in monozygotic twins is 50%.

Psychosocial Factors

Stressful life events and environmental factors play a role in the causation of mood disorders. It has been observed that these factors play a major role in the first episode rather than in the subsequent ones.

Some clinicians believe that life events play the primary or principal role in depression.

Premorbid Personality Factors

People with certain personality types–oral–defendants, obsessive–compulsive, hysterical are at a greater risk of depression.

CLINICAL FEATURES

A. DEPRESSIVE EPISODES

A depressed mood and a loss of interest or pleasure are the key symptoms of depression. Patient may have feelings of hopelessness and a general negative attitude towards self, the world and the future.

Depressed mood in a depressed patient often has a distinct quality that differentiates it from the normal emotion of sadness or grief. Almost all depressed patients complain of reduced energy and difficulty in initiating activities. Their school and work performance may be impaired.

Disturbances in sleep are common. Most patients have difficulty in initiating sleep, multiple awakenings during the night and early morning awakening (Terminal Insomnia). Depressed patients may have decreased appetite and weight loss at one end of the spectrum and some have increased appetite and weight gain at the other end.

Cognitive symptoms are experienced by some patients include subjective reports of an inability to concentrate and impairments in thinking. Anxiety is a common co morbid symptom. Other vegetative symptoms include abnormal menses and decreased interest and performance in sexual activities. Depressed patients may exhibit a whole range of somatic complaints.

Depression in Special Age Groups

1. **Children and adolescents:** School phobia and excessive clinging to parents may be symptoms of depression in children. Poor academic performance, substance abuse, antisocial behavior, sexual promiscuity, truancy and running away may be symptoms of depression in adolescents.
2. **Depression and suicide:** About 2/3 of all depressed patients contemplate suicide, and 10-15% commit suicide.

Psychotic Symptoms in Depression

Depressed patients with delusion and hallucination are said to have a major depressive episodes with psychotic features. Delusions and hallucinations that are consistent with a depressed mood like delusions of guilt, sinfulness, poverty, failure or terminal somatic illness are referred to as being mood congruent. Delusions and hallucinations that are inconsistent with the mood are referred to as being mood incongruent. In severe cases patients may have delusions of nihilism i.e. false belief that self, others or the world is non-existent or coming to an end.

Depression with Atypical Features

This category has been described in DSM IV classification. The patients with atypical features of depression have mood reactivity, significant weight gain or increase in appetite, hypersomnia, leaden paralysis i.e. heavy feeling in arms and legs and long standing pattern of interpersonal rejection sensitivity.

B. MANIC EPISODES

Manic episodes are characterized by an abnormally elevated, expansive or irritable mood. The various degree of elevated mood are:

A. **Euphoria: Stage 1:** It is a state of increased sense of well-being which is not in keeping with the environmental events. Seen in Hypomania.
B. **Elation: Stage 2:** It is a state of increased sense of wellbeing along with increased psychomotor activity. Classical of mania.
C. **Exaltation: Stage 3:** It is a stage of intense elation with delusions of grandiosity.
D. **Ecstasy: Stage 4:** It is a state of intense rapture or bliss. It is seen in delirious or stuperous mania.

Associated symptoms include, increased activity or physical restlessness, increased talkativeness, flight of ideas or the subjective experience of thought racing, loss of normal social inhibitions, resulting in behavior that is inappropriate to the circumstances, decreased need for sleep, inflated self esteem or grandiosity, distractibility or constant changes in activity or plans. These symptoms should be present for at least one week or even less if the symptoms are severe enough to require hospitalization to diagnose a manic episode. Hypomania can be distinguished from mania by its short duration (Only 4 days duration of symptoms required for a diagnosis and lesser severity of symptoms).

Mania with Psychotic Features

It is characterized by manic symptoms accompanied by hallucinations and delusions. The theme of delusion is usually grandiose. The psychotic features may be consistent with the mood (mood congruent) or inconsistent with the mood (Mood incongruent).

Bipolar Affective Disorder

This disorder (earlier known as manic depressive psychosis) is characterized by episodes of both mania and depression in the same individual at different times and not necessarily alternatively.

As per the new diagnostic guidelines (ICD – 10 and DSM IV) an individual even if he has all episodes of mania is classified as bipolar disorder. The current episode of the disorder may be hypomanic, manic, depressive (mild, moderate, severe) or mixed.

Persistent Mood Disorders

These disorders include Cyclothymia and Dysthymic disorder.

Cyclothymia: In this disorder the individual experiences episodes of hypomania and mild depression for at least a period of 2 years and the person has not been without the symptoms for more than 2 months at a time.

Dysthymic disorders: Dysthymic Disorder is a chronic disorder characterized by the presence of a depressed mood that lasts most of the day and is present on most days for a period of 2 years. Associated symptoms include feeling of inadequacy, guilt, irritability, withdrawal from society, loss of interest and lack of productivity

COURSE AND PROGNOSIS

Bipolar mood disorder has an onset in the third decade while the recurrent depressive disorder has slightly later onset. Unipolar depressive episode has a bimodal peak in the late third decade and fifth to sixth decade.

Duration of an average manic episode is 2-3 months and that of a depressive episode is 5-13 months if untreated.

However with early institution of treatment, the majority of the symptoms of mania are controlled within 2 weeks and that of depression within 4-6 weeks. Bipolar affective disorder has a better prognosis than schizophrenia but a poorer prognosis than major depressive disorder.

Good prognostic factors associated with the course of bipolar mood disorder are short duration of manic episodes, late age of onset, few coexisting psychotic or medical problems and milder nature of episodes.

Poor prognostic indicators are poor premorbid occupational status, alcohol and other substance dependence, psychotic features; inter episodic depressive features and male gender.

If a patient has 4 or more cycles of mood episodes in a year he is classified as a rapid cycler which has implications in the prognosis and choice of psychopharmacological treatment.

A patient having frequent switches and a great number of affective episodes is classified as ultra-rapid cycler.

Seasonal Pattern

Patients with seasonal pattern mood disorders tend to experience depressive episodes during a particular season, most commonly in winter. The pattern has become known as seasonal affective disorder. These patients are likely to respond to treatment with light therapy.

OTHER TYPES

Endogenous/Reactive Continuums

Endogenous/Reactive continuums is a controversial division. It implies that endogenous depressions are biological and reactive depression is psychological occurring after an identifiable stress. Other symptoms of endogenous depression have been described as diurnal variation, delirious psychomotor retardation, early morning awakening and feeling of guilt. Symptoms of reactive depression have been described as including initial insomnia, anxiety, emotional lability and multiple somatic complaints.

Double Depression

It is a condition in which major depressive disorder is superimposed on Dysthymic disorder.

MEDICAL MANAGEMENT

Treatment of mood disorders is often a rewarding experience as there is complete recovery from symptoms but nevertheless a challenging one due to frequent recurrence of symptoms. Treatment of mood disorders could be divided into:

A. Treatment of manic episode.
B. Treatment of major depressive disorder or recurrent major depressive disorder.
C. Treatment of bipolar affective disorder.

A. **Treatment of a Manic Episode:** A manic episode requires quick interventions as any delay could result in serious psychological and economic repercussions for the patient and his family. Hospitalization may be indicated for the purpose of diagnosis, the risk of suicide or homicide, history of rapidly progressive symptoms and rupture of a patient's usual support system.

The current strategy is to start a patient on a mood stabilizer along with benzodiazepines for control of agitation and insomnia. The choice of a drug depends on the clinician's preference and patients profile. Mood stabilizers generally used are lithium carbonate, Divalproex sodium and carbamazepine.

Use of Antipsychotics

Use of Antipsychotics is warranted for treatment of psychotic symptoms and for the initial few days of treatment till the mood stabilizer takes its effect. Recently atypical antipsychotics (olanzapine, risperidone, Clozapine etc.) have been evaluated for their role in treatment of acute manic episode associated with bipolar affective disorder.

B. **Treatment of Major Depressive Episode**: Most studies indicate that a combination of psychotherapy and pharmacotherapy is the most effective treatment for major depressive disorder. Psychotherapy alone may be effective for mild depressive episode but for a moderate or a severe episode pharmacotherapy should be initiated along with psychotherapy.

Psychotherapy: There are three types of short term psychotherapies (Cognitive Therapy, Interpersonal Therapy and Behavior Therapy) indicated for treatment of depression.

1. **Cognitive therapy:** This therapy developed by Aaron Beck, focuses on the cognitive distortions postulated to be present in major depressive disorder. Such distortions include selective attention to the negative aspects of circumstances and unrealistically morbid inferences. The goal of cognitive therapy is to alleviate depressive episode and to prevent their recurrence by helping patients to recognize and test negative cognition, develop alternative, flexible and positive ways of thinking and rehearse new cognitive and behavioral responses.
2. **Interpersonal therapy:** This therapy developed by Gerald Klerman focuses on one or two of patient's current interpersonal problems. This therapy is based on two assumptions; First, Current interpersonal problems are likely to have their roots in early dysfunctional relationships. Second, Current interpersonal problems are likely to be involved in precipitating or perpetuating the current depressive symptoms. The interpersonal therapy program usually consists of 12-16 weekly sessions and is characterized by an active therapeutic approach.
3. **Behavior therapy:** Behavior therapy is based on the hypothesis that maladaptive behavior patterns result in a person receiving little positive feedback, and perhaps out right rejection from society; by addressing maladaptive behaviors in therapy, patients learns to function in the world in such a way that they receive positive reinforcement.

Pharmacotherapy: Depression can be treated by a whole range of antidepressant drugs (see table).

Tricyclic
1. Imipramine
2. Amitriptyline
3. Clomipramine
4. Desipramine.

SSRIs
1. Fluoxetine
2. Paroxetine
3. Sertraline
4. Fluvoxamine

SNRIs
1. Venlafaxine
2. Duloxetine

MAOs
1. Phenelzine
2. Tranylcypromine

Others
1. Bupropion
2. Mirtazapine

Most clinicians use SSRIs as the first line treatment of major depressive disorder because of their effectiveness and favorable adverse effect profile.

Role of ECT: ECT is indicated in patients with severe depression with suicidal ideation and in those patients in which pharmacotherapy is not effective or not tolerated.

C. **Treatment of Bipolar Affective Disorder:** Lithium, Carbamazepine and divalproex are drugs commonly used for treatment and prevention of Bipolar Disorders.

Lithium carbonate: Lithium is still a standard treatment for bipolar disorder. However its side effects like; poly urea, weight gain, Tremors, Memory loss, thyroid disorders, acne, and psoriasis limit its use. Effectiveness and compliance of lithium can be monitored by measuring the level of lithium in serum. Lithium is also effective in bipolar depression. The recommended blood levels of lithium are:
Therapeutic Blood Lithium–0.8-1.2 meq/l
Prophylactic Blood lithium–0.6-1.2 meq/l.

Divalproex: Divalproex is rapidly replacing lithium as first line therapy in bipolar disorder due to its better side effect profile. Divalproex is also effective in dysphoric mania and in rapid cycling patients.

Carbamazepine: Carbamazepine is an effective alternative to lithium.

Other drugs used:

1. Clonazepam.
2. Lamotrigin.
3. Gabapentine.
4. Topiramate.
5. T_3 and T_4 are used for treatment of rapid cyclers and resistant depressions as adjuncts.

NURSING MANAGEMENT

Nursing Assessment

During assessment of a patient with mood disorder, a nurse should observe mood and affect, thinking, perception, sleep pattern and other biological functions. Patients experiencing a manic episode will likely display a bright or happy mood, while a person with depression will usually display a sad mood or flat affect with a lack of eye contact.

During mania, thoughts become faster and may become fragmented, leading to disorganized patterns of speech. Complaints of "racing thoughts" are common in people with manic episode. The person may be preoccupied with delusional thinking.

A. **Assessment of a patient with mania:** For assessment of a manic patient, emphasis should be on evaluating symptoms of mania, and most particular on change in sleep-pattern. On going assessment should focus on irritability, fatigue, and potential for harming self or others.

- Assess whether the patient is able to verbalize thoughts and feelings.
- Monitor patient's patterns of verbal speech. The tone, volume and pressure of speech spoken are all relevant. Changes in the tone and rate can provide clues to mood and energy level. Patients in a manic state have very pressured or loud and have forceful speech.
- Assess for patient's increased or decreased sleep patterns. Person with manic episode often remains sleepless for even 2 to 3 days.
- Assess the patient's energy level. Manic patient will usually report a drastic increase in energy, in contrast to depressed patient, who usually reports anergia or decreased energy levels.
- A loss of weight may be seen in a manic patient as the excessive activity minimizes the perceived need for food.
- Determine the amount of assistance required for personal hygiene, dressing, and elimination needs. Both the manic and

depressed persons may lack attention to hygiene and bowel habits.

B. **Assessment of a patient with depression:** For assessment of a depressed patient, emphasis should be on evaluating change in appetite and sleep patterns, decreases energy level, disturbances of mood and affect, thought process and contents, cognition, change in social and family relationships.

- Record sleep patterns, depressed patients usually have insomnia with difficulty in falling asleep and staying asleep.
- Assess appetite, recent eating patterns, and weight changes. Patients with depression may have little appetite or overeat as a coping tool.
- Determine the level of orientation. In depressive states, thought processes are retarded or slowed; concentration may be difficult for either the manic or depressed patient.
- Determine suicidal ideation or plan if any.
- Ask the patient about any somatic complaints. During depression, the tolerance for pain may decrease, giving rise to generalized body aches, headaches, and gastrointestinal disturbances.
- Assess need of assistance required for personal hygiene, dressing, and elimination needs. Both the manic and depressed person may lack attention to hygiene and bowel habits.

Nursing Diagnosis

Once information has been collected, the nurse identifies the individual needs of the patient. The needs of the depressed patient may be very different from those of one experiencing a manic episode.

A. Nursing diagnoses of depressive patient

Biological Domain

- Activity intolerance.
- Sleep pattern disturbance.
- Sexuality patterns altered.
- Nutrition, altered.
- Self care deficit.

Psychological Domain

- Coping, individual ineffective.
- Hopelessness.
- Violence directed at self or others.
- Low self-esteem.
- Altered family processes.

Social Domain

- Powerlessness.
- Social isolation.
- Ineffective family coping.

B. Nursing diagnoses of hypomanic or manic patient

Biological domain:

- Sleep pattern disturbance, related to inability to recognize fatigue and hyperactivity.
- Nutrition altered (less than body requirements), related to inadequate food intake and excessive activity.
- Self-care deficit, related to hyperactivity and delusional thoughts.
- Violence, self-directed or directed at others, related to irritability and delusional thinking.
- Non compliance, if patients have stopped taking their medication.

Psychological domain:

- Anxiety.
- Communication impaired.
- Coping, individual, ineffective, related to delusional ideas.
- Thought processes altered, related to delusions of grandiosity or persecution.

- Sensory/perceptual alteration, related to bizarre thinking and overload.

Social Domain:

- Family process altered.
- Impaired social interaction.
- Personal identity disturbance, related to delusional thinking.
- unrealistic perception.

Expected Outcomes

After proper assessment and formulation of nursing diagnosis, anticipated outcomes that are realistic in terms of the individual patient should be outlined. Patients are often in a severe mood state when admitted to a psychiatric facility. Stabilization is necessary before the person is able to recognize and deal with the underlying issues.

Expected Outcomes for Depressed Patient

Immediate and Long term outcomes

- Experiences decreased feelings of self-blame and doubt.
- Increased patient's energy level.
- Identifies personal strengths.
- Reframes thoughts into positive statements.
- Expresses feelings openly.
- Demonstrates improved skills to deal with loss.
- Resumes sexual functioning with partner.
- Increased interaction with others.
- Participates in unit activities every day.
- Taking adequate meal each day.
- Regularization of sleep pattern with 4 to 6 hours of sleep.
- Performs activities of daily living independently.

Expected Outcomes for the Patient of Hypomania or Mania

- Maintains self-control with decreased agitation.
- Exhibits decreased activity level.
- Takes care, meal and nutritional supplements everyday.
- Performs Activities of daily living independently.
- Receives 4 to 6 hours of uninterrupted sleep.
- Participates appropriately in unit activities.
- Interacts appropriately with others.
- Verbalizes realistic expectations of self.
- Continuous family participation in planning process.
- Channels psychologic energy into productive activity.
- Help him to maintain accurate perception of reality.

Nursing Interventions

Nursing intervention should be planned individually for each patient. All patients with an altered mood state may be very sensitive to behaviors and verbal statements of others. It is important for the nurse to plan actions that allow the person to make progress toward improved functioning and a sense of well-being. Interventions should be implemented according to priority of need.

Interventions will differ depending on the mood state the patient is experiencing.

Nursing Interventions for the Depressed Patient

- Establish a therapeutic relationship with the patient and maintain it.
- Keep a close monitoring on current depressive symptoms or development of new ones.
- Encourage him to maintain hygiene and self-care needs independently.
- Ensure that he brushes his teeth, takes his bath and performs other activities regularly.
- Ask the patient about any suicidal thoughts indicating a plan of how, when, or where the patient might harm or kill self.

- Assess the patient's energy level-as energy increases, the ability to carry out a plan for suicide increases.
- Check for sharp instruments or any other such things (collecting some drugs) that can be used for suicidal plan.
- Encourage the patient to explore feelings and communicate them in a safe manner.
- Assist the patient to express anger and other negative feelings appropriately.
- Help patient to recognize situations he or she can control and explore alternatives for those that cannot be controlled.
- Encourage the patient to recognize negative thoughts and teach reframing techniques.
- Teach alternative methods of coping with life situations that are constructive and safe.
- Focus on patient's strengths and positive attributes.
- Assist the patient in establishing realistic goals.
- Encourage the patient to participate in unit activities and assist him to perform activities of daily living as needed.
- Educate the patient regarding depression and treatment and stress on importance of taking medications as prescribed.
- Remind him of his worthiness and help him to socialize with others.
- Treatment of depression also involves combination of various therapies like Pharmacotherapy, ECT and psychotherapy. The Nurse should provide information about these therapies and also explain to him about their effects and side effects.

NURSING INTERVENTIONS FOR THE MANIC PATIENT

- Assess risk for accidents to self or others.
- Maintain calm, supportive and a safe environment.
- Decrease environmental stimuli by avoiding noises and voices.
- Observe the patient frequently and limit his behavior.
- Refrain from becoming angry with patients who are hostile or behaving in an inappropriate manner.
- Avoid arguing with or being charmed by patients.
- Convey a non reactive attitude when the patient has inappropriate behavior.
- Encourage appropriate dressing and grooming and redirect the patient when acting out in a sexual manner.
- Educate patient regarding need of medications and other treatment methods.
- Give regular medications to the patient and check for side effects, if any.
- Provide nutritional finger foods when the client is unable to sit long enough to eat.
- Monitor intake and output to prevent dehydration by providing water and juices in containers patient can carry.
- Monitor for escalating anxiety that may lead to explosive behavior.
- Spend time with the patient—if the patient is unable to sit, walk with him or her.
- Provide positive feedback when appropriate.

SPECIFIC INTERVENTIONS FOR A SUICIDAL PATIENT

On admission, patient should be assessed for various risk factors that indicate a suicide plan. Determine the content of any suicidal thoughts or ideations and lethality of the method. A more lethal method usually indicates increased likelihood of an attempt. If the patient has recently attempted suicide, continuous monitoring of the patient is indicated. The sharp and dangerous items should be removed from the patient's room. Random checks of patients are to be done to avoid possible attempt. It is also important to spend time with patient who is considering suicide as the only option. Be active listening and being present, the nurse conveys a sense of caring and appreciation for the worth of the patient.

Evaluation

Evaluation focuses improvement in patient's thought processes, behavior, and overall functioning. The effectiveness of interventions related to anxiety and coping ability will be demonstrated as the patient appropriately verbalizes feelings and thoughts. Behavior changes indicate an improvement in self-control and application of more effective coping skills. Interest and participation in self-care and hygiene show an elevation in self-appreciation. Increased hope and worth relieves the acute need for self-destruction, although an increased risk may exist for those who are showing improvement and energized enough to carry out a preconceived idea.

As anxiety reduces and excessive mood states are under control, the patient is able to eat and sleep with less disturbances. Improved communication and social interaction will result as thought processes become more rational and reality oriented. The maintenance of a continued state of mood stability will depend on compliance with the medication and follow-up treatment plan.

KEY POINTS

- Mood refers to the internal emotional state of an individual and Affect is the external expression of emotional content.
- Emil Kraepelin in 1896 first described the concept of manic depressive psychosis.
- Norepinephrine and serotonin are the two neurotransmitters, most implicated in pathophysiology of mood disorders, their levels increase in mania and decrease in depression.
- Atypical depression usually have an onset in teens and characterized by increase appetite, increase sleep, leaden paralysis and hypersensitivity to rejection.
- The lifetime prevalence for major depressive disorders is about 10-25% for woman and 5-12% for man. For bipolar affective disorder the lifetime prevalence varies from 0.4% to 1.6%.
- A depressed mood and a loss of interest or pleasure are the key symptoms of depression. Patient may have feelings of hopelessness and a general negative attitude towards self, the world and the future.
- Manic Episodes are characterized by an abnormally elevated, expansive or irritable mood with increase psychomotor activity.
- Patients with a seasonal pattern to mood disorders tend to experience depressive episodes during a particular season, most commonly in winter. This pattern is known as seasonal affective disorder. These patients are likely to respond to treatment with light therapy.
- Mood stabilizers generally used are lithium carbonate, Divalproex sodium and carbamazepine.
- The recommended blood levels of lithium for-Therapeutic Blood Lithium–0.8-1.2 meq/l and Prophylactic Blood lithium–0.6-1.2 meq/l.
- Cognitive Therapy, Interpersonal Therapy and Behavior Therapy are indicated for treatment of depression.
- SSRIs are preferred first line treatment of major depressive disorder because of their effectiveness and favorable adverse effect profile.

- Nurse must have knowledge of anti depressant medications and their therapeutic effects, associated side effects, toxicity, doses and contraindications. Patient education and provision of emotional support during the course of treatment are nurse's responsibility.
- Establishing and maintaining a therapeutic relationship is key to successful outcomes. Nursing interventions like being available in time of crisis, providing understanding and education to patient and their families, providing encouragement and feedback concerning the patient's progress and guidance in interpersonal interactions with others etc. foster the therapeutic relationship.
- Psychosocial interventions include self-care management, patient's and family education, marital and family therapy, group therapy cognitive therapy and behavior therapy.

19 Neurotic, Stress Related and Somatoform Disorders

Neuroses are the most common psychiatric disorders. These disorders include Anxiety spectrum disorders, somatoform disorders and dissociative disorders. These disorders are diagnosed only when the symptoms interfere with the patients social, occupational or personal functioning. These disorders have a myriad of causes and similar clinical picture may be obtained in a number of medical disorders. Thus one should be familiar with it.

1. ANXIETY DISORDERS

According to W.H. Auden the modern era is "age of anxiety." The current concept of civilization, the rapidity of change and partial relinquishment of religious and family values are creating new conflicts and anxieties for the individual and society.

Anxiety is a diffused, highly unpleasant, often vague feeling of apprehension, accompanied by one or more bodily sensations. Anxiety is an alerting signal; it warns of impending danger and enables the person to take measures to deal with a threat. Fear is also an alerting signal. Fear is in response to a threat that is known, external, definite or nonconflictual in origin. Anxiety is in response to a threat that is unknown, internal, vague, or conflictual in origin.

Under the heading of anxiety disorders five disorders are included: Panic disorder, phobias, generalized anxiety disorder, obsessive compulsive disorder, acute stress reaction and post traumatic Stress disorder. They have been clubbed together because anxiety is the common feature among all of them, i.e., they induce intense anxiety in the patients. They are also biochemically similar and thus they respond to similar drugs. We will discuss each disorder in brief.

A. Panic Disorder

A panic attack described as sudden onset of intense anxiety in the patients. Patients feel all the symptoms of sympathetic stimulation e.g., palpitations, tachycardia, sweating, tremors, hypertension, diarrhea or abdominal disturbance. He appears frightened and pupils are wide. Symptoms may or may not have the precipitating factors. Symptoms start without warning and usually subside by themselves after 10-15 minutes. Such panic attacks commonly occur twice weekly. Panic disorder can occur at any age, but typically have an onset between late adolescence and mid 30s. The lifetime prevalence of panic disorders is approximately two percent of the population. Panic disorder is diagnosed only when patients have the persistent concern for the symptoms. We must appreciate this important difference. ICD-10 has prescribed following features for the diagnosis.

Psychological symptoms	Autonomic symptoms
• An intense fear and feeling that they are not going to survive, • Feel that they are going to become crazy	Autonomic symptoms palpitation, choking sensation, chest pain, dizziness, vertigo or unsteady feelings Abdominal symptoms like feeling
• Fear that they are going to have heart attack or respiratory failure	of sinking in the pit of stomach, diarrhoea, motor tension, restlessness, frequency of micturation, sweaty cold and clammy limbs.
• Severe apprehension and anxiety.	These symptoms develop within minutes and reach their peak between 10-15 minutes and usually subside within an hour.

It is commonly found with Agoraphobia that involves fear of those places from where escape might be difficult viz., crowded places, bridge, motor vehicle ,closed room etc. More than 95% of those diagnosed with agoraphobia have an accompanying diagnosis of panic disorder.

Differential Diagnosis

Thyrotoxicosis, Pheochromocytoma, Mitral valve prolapse, Paroxysmal supraventricular tachycardia, asthma must be excluded before starting treatment.

Treatment

Treatment can be pharmacological or non pharmacological.

In *pharmacological treatment* we can use benzodiazepines.

However, the most prescribed drugs are SSRIs. Since they are themselves anxiogenic in short term effect, they should be prescribed in low doses. Remember the dictum ¨C start low, go slow, that means their doses should be slowly escalated. Efficacy is similar with both the group of drugs.

The beta blockers like propanolol, atenolol are particularly useful in management of anticipatory anxiety.

Non pharmacological treatments include Cognitive behavior therapy, hyperventilation control, relaxation exercises, interoceptive exposure etc.

For best outcome it is better to combine both the treatments.

B. Phobia

It involves experience of intense, persistent, irrational and recurrent fear about a particular object, place or situation that results in compelling desire to avoid the action or situation. The subject himself understands and explains the presence of fear that is interfering with his performance. Often he is unable to provide any clue regarding its genesis. Phobias are sub classified as follows-

Agora phobia: Agoraphobia is fear of those spaces from where escape might be impossible to a safe place.

Social phobia: In social phobia, subject is unable to face the people. He fears that they would be scrutinizing his actions, his way of dressing, the manner he eats, he talks etc. Due to it he becomes unable to talk to people, leaves using public lavatories, does not eat in social gatherings etc. Typical occasions where this phobia occurs are social activities and occasions where a person will be speaking, dining or writing in public. Although person recognizes the fear as unrealistic, and tries to overcome the anxiety by using drugs or alcohol.

Specific phobia: These include all other situations which are not covered either in agoraphobia or social phobias. If it involves the closed spaces it is known as Claustrophobia, Acrophobia is the fear of heights. Similarly other common phobic situations are darkness, blood, particular animals like lizards, worms etc.

Alcohol and drug dependence and major depressive disorders are the common associated conditions with phobic disorders.

Differential Diagnosis

Panic disorder can be excluded by presence of discrete episodes and focus of concern, post traumatic stress disorder must be excluded by history.

Treatment

Drugs of choice are SSRIs, though all the antidepressants are effective. Benzodiazepines are used as adjunctive measures. Specific behavior therapy involves graded exposure and response prevention, flooding and relaxation technique.

C. Generalized Anxiety Disorders (GAD)

It is the most common psychiatric disorder in general population with one year prevalence of 3-8%. Patient presents with persistent anxiety and worries for 6 months that affect number of activities of person's life. He has difficulty in controlling these.

They are expressed as palpitations, numbness, breathlessness, chest pain, discomfort, dizziness, unsteadiness, sweating, trembling, shaking or tremors, abdominal discomfort, diarrhea, excessive thirst, frequency of micturition, difficulty in concentration, intense fear or terror often associated with feelings of impending doom (or death) or loosing control, irritability, muscle tension, easy fatigability or sleep disturbances. The symptoms cause marked impairment in patient's overall functioning.

Differential Diagnosis

The syndrome must be differentiated from depression, dysthymia and other anxiety disorders. Care should be taken to rule out cardiovascular disorders, thyroid disorders, carcinoids, cushings, substance withdrawal syndromes, respiratory disorders and metabolic disorders.

Treatment

Patient should be started with SSRIs (Escitalopram, Paroxetine, Fluoxetine, and sertraline), SNRIs (Venlaflaxine) or Non sedating TCAs, (Trazodone, Imipramine). Drug should be started in low doses. If patient does not respond, benzodiazepines (Alprazolam, Clonazepam) may be added. If patient still does not improve, antidepressants should be discontinued and buspirone should be added. Buspirone is a new Antianxiety drug which does not have any dependence potential like benzodiazepines. It takes 2-3 weeks before its action is apparent.

Psychological treatments include cognitive behavior Therapy and relaxation techniques like Jacobson's progressive relaxation technique, self hypnosis and meditation.

D. Obsessive Compulsive Disorder (OCD)

This is an intriguing and often debilitating syndrome characterized by presence of two distinct phenomena: Obsession and Compulsions.

Obsessions are intrusive, unwanted, recurrent ideas, images, or impulses that hit the subject's consciousness and are ego dystonic. They are difficult to dismiss. Compulsions are repetitive behavior that can be mental or observable, done in order to reduce the anxiety produced by the obsession. Usually both occur together, but any of them may occur independently also. Obsessions may involve pathological doubts, contamination (most common), symmetry, aggressive, sexual thoughts etc. Similarly compulsions can be checking, washing, symmetry and precision, counting or hoarding. Multiple obsession or compulsions may also be present.

Epidemiology

Recent studies show the life time prevalence of OCD is as high as 2-3%. Among adults, men and women are equally affected.

Differential Diagnosis

They should be differentiated from other anxiety disorders, psychosis (by presence of other features e.g. delusions, hallucinations), touretts syndrome (difficult to differentiate), impulse control disorders, hypochondriasis (main concern with the body, not ego dystonic), and body dysmorphic disorder (Not ego dystonic).

Treatment

Pharmacotherapy: The SSRIs, especially Fluoxetine and Fluovoxamine have been described to be helpful and marketed as anti obsessional drugs, while the paroxetine and sertraline are also effective in some patients. They must be given in high doses for prolonged periods (a few weeks to a few years). Clomipramine was the first drug used effectively in the treatment of OCD and still has a special place in the treatment.

Behavioral therapy: Behavior modification is an effective mode of therapy for OCD. Behavioral therapies include graded exposure, response prevention, thought stopping and modeling (see chapter 25).

Course and outcome: About half the patients have the onset in childhood and it takes about 5-10 years before the patient receives medical treatment. The follow up studies show that one third patients recover well, while half have moderate improvement and remaining have deteriorating course.

E. Post-Traumatic Stress Disorder (PTSD)

This disorder arises in a person after witnessing a catastrophic trauma (Disasters, War, Rape, Accidents etc). After trauma patients often suffer from recollection of the thoughts and/or images of the trauma followed by intense anxiety symptoms. They may occur as disturbing dreams and trauma is re-experienced (*flashbacks*). Patients usually avoid the situation, in which they met trauma (*avoidance*) and do not like to talk about it. If the time lapse is less than one month it is termed as acute stress reaction and if it lasts more than one month after the traumatic episode it is called PTSD.

Differential Diagnosis

Must be differentiated from panic disorder, Phobia and OCD.

Treatment

Antidepressants are the mainstay of treatment. Among them, SSRIs are most commonly prescribed. They have advantage of good efficacy with minimal adverse effects. However, if arousal symptoms are the prominent part of the clinical picture, benzodiazepines can be added.

Disaster management is very important and effective measure to provide speedy help and to prevent disability. Cognitive behavior therapy and psychodynamic therapy are also helpful.

NURSING MANAGEMENT OF ANXIETY DISORDER

When establishing a nurse-patient relationship with the person experiencing excessive anxiety, it is important to initially take steps to lower the anxiety level. The nurse can best encourage the patient to come out with his problem by a calm and reassuring approach.

Nursing Assessment

For assessment of the patient with anxiety disorders, the nurse should first make observations of basic characteristics of the patient such as thought processes, affect, communication and psychomotor activity. The nurse should use directive questions to elicit subjective information about how the patient is currently feeling and what happened before the onset of symptoms. Leading Statements such as: Tell me what happened? Tell me details of what happened? How did you feel at that time? What were you thinking when that happened? What emotions were you feeling at that particular time? What are you doing to decrease that feeling? Tell me more about that? Encourage the patient participation.

Ask the patient about other somatic symptoms such as fatigue, muscle aches, eating patterns, bowel habits, sleeping patterns and fatigue that might further indicate a psychological origin for the complaints. Observe the patient during activities of daily living. Assessing the patient during usual activities can also provide clues about the patient's thought processes. Things may not mean much to others, but they may be very meaningful to the patients.

Similarly patient's affect, his ability to communicate thought,his capabilities to perform and complete tasks and psychomotor activity level should be observed by nurse.

During interaction with patient nurse must also be aware of his or her own verbal and non-verbal messages. Anxiety is contagious and can contribute to the patient's difficulty in communicating.

Observation of patient with attention to specific anxiety reducing behaviors should be part of initial and ongoing assessment for each patient. Sometimes symptoms are expressed in subtle ways, such as leaving group activity to go to bathroom or avoiding an activity where several patients are participating. It is important to note if behaviors are improving with administration of anti-anxiety medications. An observation for side-effects is also a nursing responsibility.

Nursing Diagnosis

Once the assessment is made and informations are collected, nurse can formulate applicable nursing diagnoses. Important and relevant nursing diagnoses for the patient with an anxiety disorder may include:

- Anxiety.
- Ineffective individual coping.
- Fear, related to extreme and unrealistic perceptions.
- Powerlessness, (related to lack of control over anxiety).
- Risk for harm directed at self or others, related to reoccurring intrusive thoughts.
- Sleep pattern disturbance.
- Social isolation, related to feeling of guilt or emotional numbness.
- Ineffective family related to situational crisis.
- Skin integrity, impaired, related to compulsive repetitive behaviour.
- Self esteem disturbance, related to feelings of inadequacy.
- Thought processes disturbed.

Expected Outcomes

When proper nursing diagnosis are made, appropriate outcomes for patients can be determined. Careful consideration should be given to a realistic time frame in which the outcomes can be achieved. Outcomes are always patient centered and time limited. Examples of outcomes may include that within 7 days, the patient will:

- Identify initial signs and symptoms of anxiety.
- Demonstrate effective strategies to lower anxiety.
- Experience increased energy.
- Look at pictures of a phobic stimulus without excessive anxiety.
- Ventilate anxiety appropriately and safely to others.
- Experience improved sleep pattern.

Similarly in long term the patient will:

- Demonstrate improved impulse control.
- Demonstrate decreased cleaning rituals.
- Identify effective coping methods to use when anxiety begins to occur.
- Identify alternative coping methods that decrease social isolation.
- Participate in small group discussions with decreased anxiety.
- Carry out normal daily living and social activities outside the house.

Nursing Interventions

While dealing with anxiety in patients, the nurse should take into consideration his or her own anxiety level and how it may affect nursing care. Subtle behaviour such as a change in the tone of voice, rushed movements or spending less time with the patient can communicate the nurse's anxiety to the patient. Establishing a sense of trust includes an ability to maintain a calm and supportive environment in which the patient feels a sense of safety and security.

When planning interventions, the nurse must remember that interventions should be timely, patient centered and realistic. The nurse should plan only what the patient is able to do at that time. Overwhelming the patients with unrealistic expectations may indicate increased anxiety in the nurse and counter productive results in the patient. Assessing the patient's tolerance for changes is essential for planning appropriate patient centered nursing interventions. Every effort should be made to assist the patient in identifying the issues that precipitate the feelings of anxiety. Assessing the behavior exhibited by the patient to a particular situation can help the patient to develop an awareness of feelings that precede the anxiety attacks. The nurse can also help the patient to try new, more adaptive coping strategies.

Such as:

- Encourage patient's participation in social interaction and exercise activities.
- Give positive reinforcement for the patient's effort to participate.
- Use a calm, reassuring approach, encourage verbalization of feeling, perception and fears.
- Identify periods of time when anxiety level is at its highest.
- Teach him how to perform stress-management techniques (progressive relaxation, music therapy, deep-breathing).
- Assist the patient with compulsive behaviors to find ways to set limits on the rituals.
- Acknowledge the behaviors but do not focus on them–it is important to express an empathetic response rather than criticize the behavior. For example, in response to a patient who has shampooed her hair 4 times in 2 hours, the nurse might say, "I am sure your scalp is getting sore from washing your hair so much", rather than, "You only need to wash your hair once a day."
- Administer antianxiety medications.
- Provide explanations regarding medications and side-effects to patient and family.
- Avoid giving advice to patient.
- Provide patient education regarding and precipitating factors.

Evaluation

At the end of the time-frame that was set to reach patient outcomes, evaluation of nursing care plan occurs. Effectiveness of interventions can be seen in the patient's ability to recognize and deal with anxiety producing factors. Once the patient identifies the relationship between unreasonable thoughts and subsequent behaviors, it is more realistic to anticipate the use of more effective coping strategies to reduce his/her anxiety. It is important for the patients to openly express the feelings and thoughts related to the situation. The effectiveness is shown when the patient reports that the anxiety has been reduced to a manageable level.

KEY POINTS

- Neurosis is most common of all psychiatric illness.
- Generalized anxiety disorders are most common neurotic disorders found across the globe.
- Panic attack is manifest by sudden onset and intense anxiety, fear or terror and often associated with feeling of impending doom.
- Patients with panic disorder are often seen in a number of health care setting , frequently in hospital emergency room or clinics, presenting with a confusing array of physical and emotional symptoms and require a skillful assessment.
- Phobia is irrational fear and specific object, situation or place resulting the avoidance of such conditions.
- Agoraphobia is most commonly seen phobia in clinical practice.
- Obsessions are persistent, recurrent ideas or thoughts or images that come in patient's mind against his will or wishes. The commonest form of obsession is thought of contamination. Compulsions are repetitive, purposeless behavior that is performed to calm down the anxiety developed out of obsessive thoughts. The most common form of compulsion is washing.
- Drugs of choice for OCD are fluvoxamine, Fluoxetine (SSRIs) and Clomipramine (TCA).
- Psycho education is important in the management of anxiety disorders and help the patient to control and cope with the anxiety reactions. It also includes education regarding medication side effects and their management.
- Thought stopping and response prevention are commonly used behavior therapy techniques for OCD.
- Behavior therapy is useful for management of phobia.
- Nurses can be instrumental in crisis intervention, medication management ,and psychoeducation.

2. SOMATOFORM DISORDERS

Somatization is the term used when unexplained physical symptoms are present that are related to psychological distress. These are a group of disorders in which the main concern of a subject is his own body. In these disorders subject complains of bodily symptoms that are often vague in nature and for which no medical explanation can be found. Patients consult doctors repeatedly, but despite persistent reassurance symptoms persist. It includes five disorders-Somatization disorder, Undifferentiated somatoform disorder, Persistent pain disorder, Hypochondriasis and Body dysmorphic disorder.

A. Somatization Disorder

Patient presents with multiple somatic complaints involving nervous system, Gastro-intestinal tract, genitourinary system, and recurring pains. Onset is almost always before 30 years and the main concern of the patient is symptoms. Disorder interferes with the functioning. Patient usually consults the physician who often fails to find out any abnormality. Symptoms should not be explained by any substance use and must not be intentionally produced. Disorder runs a fluctuating course with occasional recurrences.

Somatization disorder was first known as hysteria. It was also called *Briquet's syndrome*. It is much commoner in women (1-2% of all female) and tends to run in families.

Differential Diagnosis

It is important to differentiate them from a variety of causes including migraine, temporal arteritis, peptic ulcer, angina, fibromyalgia, myasthenia, diabetic neuropathy, irritable bowel syndrome, stroke, epilepsy etc. Besides medical disorder it must be excluded from OCD, other somatoform disorders, persistent delusional disorder, dissociative disorders and depression with somatic features.

Treatment

Psychotherapy is helpful for patients with Somatization disorders. The main concern is to decrease the sick role by double bind messages and avoiding unnecessary investigations. Patient must be educated regarding disease. For proper management strong therapeutic relationship is required, otherwise patient may turn hostile. Third step is reassurance regarding the benign nature of symptoms. His interpersonal issues that aggravate the symptoms must be gradually explored and treated. Pharmacotherapy is not very effective. It should be directed to the treatment of associated anxiety and depression. Antidepressants might be of help in some patients, but benzodiazepine must be used with caution in light of addiction potential.

B. Undifferentiated Somatoform Disorder

It is diagnosed when patient presents with one or more somatic complaint which can not be explained by the medical cause despite careful investigations and are not the result of substance use. If the complaints co-occur with medical disorder then patient's preoccupation is more than desired. It must impair the functioning of person and persist for at least 6 months. These are those patients who do not meet criterion for somatization disorder.

Differential Diagnosis

It must be carefully differentiated from the medical and surgical disorders of affected system that may simulate.

Treatment

Treatment principles are the same as described for somatization disorder.

C. Persistent Pain Disorder

Pain at one or more anatomical sites is the predominant focus of attention that causes significant distress in social, occupational or other areas of functioning. The physician must be sure that psychological factors are playing an important part in production and maintenance of symptoms. This can be diagnosed even when the medical cause of pain is apparent, provided pain complained by the patient is excessive to one, which can be induced by medical disorder. ICD 10 requires the persistence of pain for at least 3 months.

Differential Diagnosis

It should be differentiated from the possible medical causes of pain. Care must be taken to exclude other somatoform disorders, depression, psychosis, substance withdrawal especially opioid withdrawal and dissociative sensory disorder.

Treatment

Most of the patients with this disorder refuse for psychiatric help. A supporting relationship with doctor is helpful. Underlying disorder whether medical or psychological must be addressed. SSRIs for long term treatment and analgesics for short term treatment can be given. Cognitive behavior therapy is also helpful.

D. Hypochondriasis

In this syndrome patient presents with fear of having some serious disease based upon the misinterpretation of normal body functions e.g., he may misinterpret normal gurgling sounds of stomach for the signs of stomach cancer. He often visits the physicians and despite their reassurance, keeps on taking advice. Most of the time when patient comes to psychiatrist, he carries a plethora of prescriptions and investigation reports with him. The condition causes malfunctioning in the patients life. For diagnosis, behavior must be present for at least 6 months, but this belief is not so fixed that it is a delusion. In general medical practice, hypochondriasis is present in 3-14% of patients. The prevalence in general population is not known. It is found equally in men and women and peak incidence occurs in fourth or fifth decade.

Differential Diagnosis

This should be differentiated from OCD, Monosymptomatic hypochondriacal delusions, Body dysmorphic disorder, depression and anxiety spectrum disorders.

Treatment

Hypochondriacs are usually resistant to psychiatric treatment. Among such patients *Group psychotherapy* has been reported to be the modality of choice. Other treatment principles are the same as in other somatoform disorders.

E. Body Dysmorphic Disorder

It is also known as "Dysmorphophobia". In this disorder, patients suffer from an imagined defect in appearance. If defect is present, then concern is markedly excessive. As for other psychiatric disorders, it also interferes with the functioning of the patient. The person may present as complaint of disfigured nose, face, breasts or genitals and may take repeated consultations from plastic surgeons and even may undergo repeated surgeries.

Differential Diagnosis

It should be differentiated from other disorders of the same group, malingering, factitious disorder, OCD, depression, schizophrenia and the anorexia nervosa.

Treatment

Cognitive behavior therapy has shown some result. Biological treatments include TCAs and MAOIs. However, SSPIs in high doses appear to benefit in delusional as well as non delusional parts of disorder. They must be combined with antipsychotics, especially Pimozide.

3. FACTITIOUS DISORDERS (*Manchausen syndrome*)

This group involves those disorders in which medical or psychiatric symptoms are intentionally produced, but only to assume sick role. Patient does not intend to feign the illness for any gain, be it monetary or otherwise.

This group has two disorders: Factitious disorder and Factitious disorder by proxy. Factitious disorder can further be classified into those: (i) with predominantly physical symptoms (*munchausen's syndrome*) e.g., fever, pain abdomen, anemia, epilepsy etc., (ii) with predominantly psychological symptoms e.g., Depression, Anxiety, Psychosis etc., and (iii) with symptoms from both categories.

In factitious disorder by proxy, the perpetrator creates the sick role in dependent person, e.g., mothers repeatedly seek advice for the illness of their baby. They may give substances that produce the symptoms mimicking some disorder in their babies. Diagnosis requires great deal of suspicion and supportive confrontation with the information, unfolded by the informant.

Etiology

Abnormalities in childhood developmental stages may also contribute to the illness. Serious childhood illnesses when combined with family dysfunctions, past anger with medical profession, past significant relationship with health care provider and factitious disorder in parent are risk factors. According to psychodynamic theory important defense mechanisms are repression, identification, identification with aggressor, regression and symbolization. It has been found that these patients suffer from a number of CNS abnormalities that can be seen on CT and MRI scanning.

Differential Diagnosis

This must be carefully differentiated from somatoform disorders in which symptom production is unconscious for unconscious psychological benefits. This must also be differentiated from malingering in which illness is feigned for some conscious benefits.

Treatment

The prognosis is very poor and treatment is mostly unsuccessful. Supportive confrontation appears to have some role. Long term psychotherapies may also benefit. Data regarding pharmacotherapy is not available.

APPLICATION OF THE NURSING PROCESS

Because the somatoform disorders are presented with physical symptoms, the person is often seen by a physician for complaints. Diagnosis testing are necessary to rule out any underlying organic pathology. It is of major importance that nursing observations and data collection contains information that will be of help in this process. Nurse must consider the fact that the patient is unaware of underlying psychological issues and is unable to control the symptoms. Most of them are repeat users of health care system services, both outpatient and inpatient.

Nursing Assessment

Nurse should try to create an accepting, safe, and supportive atmosphere that allows open communication with the patient and his or her family. Then nurse should focus on the whole person, including psycho logic, social, and family factors in addition to the physical symptoms.

After careful assessment of physical complaints nurse must note any preoccupation with the symptoms and any inconsistency between what is being described and what is observed in the patient. It is important to note the patient's attitude toward the symptoms and how he or she may view any limitations caused by them. It should also be noted whether the patient is aware of events surrounding the onset of symptoms. In addition, the patient's level of anxiety and his coping skills should be assessed.

Nursing Diagnosis

Nursing care plan for the patient with a somatoform disorder must consider that the patient is often frustrated and irritated by the implication that the symptoms are psychologic. Nursing diagnoses to these disorders may include:

- Chronic pain, related to severe anxiety or unmet dependency needs.
- Sleep pattern disturbance, related to anxiety, depression, or chronic pain.
- Sexual dysfunction, related perceived loss of body function or fear of contracting major disease.

- Anxiety, severe, related to repressed trauma or unmet dependency needs.
- Ineffective coping, related to anxiety, repression, or unrealistic perceptions.
- Social isolation, related preoccupation with self and chronic state of perceived illness.
- Knowledge deficit, related to psychophysiology nature of illness.
- Ineffective treatment regimen management.
- Self-esteem disturbance, related to repressed unmet dependency needs and unsatisfactory interpersonal relationships.

Expected Outcomes

Once problems have been identified for the individual patient's situation, planning will include realistic outcomes in the course of treatment:

- Acknowledges that physical pain may be associated with psycho logic stress.
- Participates in development of a plan for effective pain control.
- Verbalizes realistic perception of minor body defect and related positive feelings.
- Verbalizes understanding of psychological factors associated with alteration in physical functioning.
- Reports a decrease in sleep-related problems.
- Expresses feelings of anxiety and effective means of dealing with the illness.
- Acknowledges understanding and perception of present health problem.
- Discusses present health problem with health care provider and family.
- Demonstrates reduced use of manipulative behavior to secure attention.
- Participates in social activities and interaction without discomfort.
- Identifies need to increase self esteem and participates in individual and group therapy for esteem building.

Nursing Interventions

Establishing a trusting relationship with patients experiencing a somatoform disorder is the first step in helping them overcome a low self-concept. A safe and supportive environment will also help lower their anxiety to a level that allows expression of underlying feelings. It must be remembered that they are not consciously trying to be sick or avoid responsibilities. Other interventions may include:

- Recognize that physical complaints are real to the client even though supportive medical evidence is lacking.
- Avoid any confrontation concerning the psychologic nature of their symptoms.
- Respond to patient with understanding and patience.
- Encourage patient to discuss various somatic problems, but allow some time to discuss psychological and interpersonal issues.
- Explore opportunities for patient to meet other people with similar problems.
- Clarify the purpose of taking medication and educate about the effects of medication.
- Identify unfulfilled dependency needs of the patient.
- Identify types of primary and secondary gain achieved by symptoms.
- Help the patient to use words rather than physical means to express feelings.
- Encourage patient to keep a diary of daily happenings and feelings, along with physical symptoms.
- Listen carefully to determine what the patient may be omitting when describing the symptoms.
- Encourage the patient to make decision and take responsibility for situations related to them.

- Help the patient to identify more effective coping mechanism rather than the somatic symptoms.

Evaluation

Evaluation of implemented nursing actions focuses on the patient's ability to recognize the underlying psychologic stress and anxiety that are contributing to the physical symptoms. Once the patient can look realistically at the connection between repressed emotional turmoil and the somatic symptoms, a decrease in complaints or full recovery from the previous level of altered physical functioning, pain, or preoccupation with body appearance is anticipated.

KEY POINTS

- Somatoform disorders are more common among females.
- Somatization disorder is characterized by presence of recurrent and multiple somatic complaints of several years duration for which medical attention is sought but which are apparently not due to any physical disorder.
- Hypochondriasis is an unrealistic interpretation of physical sign or sensations as abnormal leading to preoccupation with the fear or belief of having a serious disease.
- Hospitalizations, investigations and medications with addictive potential should be avoided in hypochondriasis.
- Psychogenic pain disorder is characterized by predominant complaint of pain without any physical or any other mental disorder.
- Psychogenic pain disorder is common in males and leads to excessive use of analgesic, request of surgery and the assumption of an invalid role.
- Patients with body Dysmorphic disorder believe that they are physically misshapen or defective in some way. Such patients do not hold this belief with the conviction of a delusion. Some persons persist in seeking plastic surgery to correct deformity.
- Identifying and diagnosing somatoform and factitious disorder is very complex because the patient with these disorders refuse to accept any psychiatric basis of their problems and often go for years moving from one health care provider to another.
- Development of the nurse-patient relationship is crucial to assessing these patients and identifying appropriate diagnosis and interventions.
- Health teaching is important in helping the individual develop positive life style changes in place of somatization responses.
- Factitious disorders are characterized by voluntary production of physical or psychological symptoms.
- Cardinal feature of Munchausen's syndrome is the attainment of the role of the patient and the motivation is not clear.
- Munchausen's syndrome is factitious disorder with physical symptoms whereas Ganser's syndrome is factitious disorder with psychological symptoms.
- Psychotherapy is treatment of choice in Munchausen's syndrome and Ganser's syndrome.

4. DISSOCIATIVE (CONVERSION) DISORDERS

Dissociation is a process that allows our mind to separate certain memories from the conscious awareness. These separated parts are kept in unconscious and are repressed. It may re-emerge, when we encounter a situation similar to original trauma. The common theme in all disorders of the group is partial or complete loss of normal integration between memories of past, awareness of identity, immediate sensations, and control of body movements, so that some part of these functions is lost. Course is usually episodic. Symptoms start suddenly and in the same manner terminate suddenly. Symptoms involve mental phenomenon. ICD-10 place following disorders in this group: (i) Dissociative amnesia, (ii) Dissociative fugue, (iii) Trance and possession syndrome, (iv) Dissociative motor disorder, (v) Dissociative sensory disorder, (vi) Dissociative convulsions, (vii) Mixed Dissociative Disorders, and (viii) other dissociative disorders that include Gansers Syndrome and Multiple Personality Disorder.

One important things to remember is that iv, v, vi and vii disorders from the above list are also commonly known as Hysteria or Conversion Reaction (CR). Reader must not be confused regarding distinction among all of them. Because of predominant involvement of physical symptoms, DSM- IV has placed it in the category of Somatoform Disorders, while due to episodic course, ICD-10 has placed it in dissociative disorders.

A. Dissociative Amnesia

This is the most common clinical type of dissociative disorder. Dissociative amnesia is characterized by an inability to remember important personal information, usually of traumatic or stressful situation. This lack of recall includes a loss of information beyond ordinary forgetfulness. The loss is reversible, unlike dementia. Loss usually follows a traumatic event, and patient is unable to recall the event. It is common in 3rd and 4th decade, and in female more than in male. The amnesia may take one of the several forms

1. **Localized amnesia:** Most common type, Loss of memory for the events of a short period of time. This acute form is more common in response to war combat, natural disasters or severe trauma.
2. **Generalized amnesia:** Loss of memory for a whole life time experience.
3. **Selective amnesia:** Failure to recall some portion of events, but not all during a short period of time.
4. **Continuous amnesia:** Forgetting each successive event as it occurs.

Before diagnosing it all possible medical causes viz. stroke, Wernickes encephalopathy and substance use disorders must be excluded.

B. Dissociative Fugue

It involves one or more episode of sudden, unexpected, purposeful travel away from home, with the inability to recall own biographical details and usually assumption of new identities. The onset is usually sudden, often in presence of severe stress. All the possible medical causes e.g., epileptic fugue, complex partial seizure and substance use must be excluded before diagnosis.

C. Trance and Possession Syndrome

In trance, there is temporary marked alteration in the state of consciousness associated with narrowing of awareness of immediate surroundings and stereotyped behaviors. In our country it can be seen in people engaged in worships at religious places who sometimes become oblivious of the surroundings and lose their social inhibitions and start performing rituals such as chant religious songs, dancing etc. When asked later they report as that they felt if they were in some other world.

In possession trance, above symptoms are followed by replacement of person's identity by some spirit. This is common in our country. Later on person is amnesic for the event.

All the possible medical disorders and substance use must be ruled out before diagnosis.

D. Dissociative Motor/Sensory/ Convulsion/Mixed Disorders (Conversion Disorders)

The term Hysteria was earlier used for conversion disorders. In this disorder person suffers from episodic loss of movement of involuntary movements, convulsions simulating epileptic fits, paresthesia or anesthesia or a mixture of all of above, which results from a psychological conflict or need.

The onset of symptom is acute and terminates after some time. They are usually followed by stress and patient may have la bella indifference i.e., calm acceptance of the serious symptoms. Patient often develop symptoms in presence of others, and usually has seen the same symptoms in the past.

In some survey the life time incidence of conversion symptoms are as high as 25-33 percent. It is 2.5 times more common in women. Adolescent girls are most often affected.

Common symptoms seen in conversion disorder are sensory symptoms, motor symptoms, and/or convulsions (see table).

Clinical presentation of conversion disorder

Sensory symptoms: Anesthesia and paraesthesia especially of the extremities, Conversion symptoms may involve the organs of special sense, producing deafness, blindness and tunnel vision. These symptoms may be unilateral or bilateral.

Motor symptoms: Motor symptoms include abnormal movements, gait disturbance, weaknesses, and paralysis. These movements generally worsen when attention is called to them. But these patient rarely fall, and if they do, they are generally not injured. Convulsive like movements are also sometimes seen. Other common Motor disturbances are paralysis and presis, involving one, two or all four limbs.

Convulsions (Hysterical Fits): Earlier known as 'hysterical fits' or pseudoseizures. It is characterized by convulsive movements and partial loss of consciousness. It is a very common disorder. Differential diagnosis with true seizures is important.

Etiology

Differential Diagnosis

Studies have found that nearly 1/3 patients suffer from pure psychological base, another 1/3 suffer from medical illness that is discovered at later stages and last 1/3 have components of both. All the possible medical disorders must be aggressively ruled out at the outset.

E. Multiple Personality Disorder

At least two or more personality states take the control of person's behavior in episodic manner. In all the states, person behaves differently, may have different characteristics and skills. All the personalities are usually not aware of each other. Transition from one personality to another usually follows trauma and may be sudden.

Psychotherapy often facilitated with thiopental sodium and hypnosis has been commonly used. This is usually a treatments refractory condition.

F. Ganser's Syndrome

It is also known as syndrome of approximate answers (*vorbeireden*). This is common in prison inmates. Person when asked to name a pen may call it pencil.

NURSING PROCESS IN DISSOCIATIVE DISORDERS

Nursing Assessment

Initially any physical condition that could produce the symptoms of amnesia and dissociation must be ruled out. These conditions include head injury, epilepsy, brain diseases, pharmacologic side effects, or substance abuse. A clinical interview for ascertaining any significant childhood or adult trauma must be conducted. Along with a physical assessment, a baseline psychosocial assessment should be done to determine behavioral alternations such as disorientation, level of anxiety, amnesia, any depression, and the extent to which functioning in the social and work environment is affected.

Nursing Diagnosis

Once assessment data are obtained, nursing diagnoses can be established in patients with dissociate disorders. Important nursing diagnosis are:

- Self-care deficit, related to mechanical trance like state or aimless wandering.
- Sensory perceptual alteration, related depersonalization and view of self.
- Personality identify disturbance, related to childhood trauma or more than one personality state.
- Altered thought processes, related to memory and repressed trauma.
- Ineffective individual coping, related to repressed memories and issues, loss of identity, or travel away from home.
- Anxiety, related to repressed traumatic events or loss of identity.
- Family coping ineffective, related to loss of identity.
- Impaired social interactions.
- Ineffective therapeutic regimen management.

Expected Outcomes

Goal of the therapeutic process is to help the person to integrate the fragmented personalities into one identity. The timeframe anticipated for symptom resolution depends upon type of dissociative disorder. Expected outcomes for the patient may include:

- Recovers memory deficits and develop improved coping mechanisms to deal with stressful events.
- Verbalizes reality-based perception of environmental stimuli in stressful situations.
- Verbalizes understanding of multipersonality states and the need to consolidate all the personalities into one.
- Performs self-care activities independently.
- Verbalizes feelings and identify positive effective ways of managing anxiety and fear.
- Self-control over behaviors toward self and others.

Nursing Interventions

The nurse must first establish a trusting and supportive therapeutic relationship with the patient. It is important to use active listening and communication techniques that encourage verbalization of feelings, conflicts, and information regarding the traumatic events that led to the current dissociative state. This process assists the patient to develop personal insight and an awareness and understanding of the self. Patients need continuous encouragement and support to achieve control over their anxiety and dissociative responses. Number of other interventions include:

- Encourage the patient to keep a daily account of thoughts and feelings.
- Develop a liaisoning between the patient and staff for dealing with self-destructive behaviors.
- Promote a safe environment to protect the patient from self-injury or injury to others.
- Assist him in developing effective coping skills.
- Model positive and desired behaviors.
- Decrease anxiety-producing stimuli.
- Use stimuli that stimulate pleasant memories and pleasurable feelings for the patient. This assists the patient to remember past experiences without the risk of precipitating increased trauma.

- Avoid flooding the patient with details of past traumatic events. This may cause the patient to regress further into the dissociative state.
- Maintain an awareness of behavioral changes that may indicate self-destructive behavior.
- Assist the patient to identify alternatives to self-injury such as regular physical exercise, written methods of expression (daily diary writing), or creative art and task-oriented activities, which provide a means of nonverbal expression of thoughts.
- Assist him to identify the purpose that each sub personality (dissociative identity disorder) serves in the total personality of the person.
- Identify contributing factors within the family dynamics and the environment.

Evaluation

In process of evaluation, progress of patient must be assessed regarding identifying and demonstrating a more adaptive response to stressful stimuli. This step helps in decreasing the dissociative response. The patient should also understand the relationship between the dissociative state and the increased anxiety. Recalling past traumatic events is crucial to this understanding in dissociative identity disorder. The evaluation process focuses on the patient's acknowledgment of the existence of more than one personality and how these various states function as protection from the anxiety related to traumatic memories. It is also important to note patient's progress towards the ultimate goal off integrating all personalities into a single personality.

Providing a safe and trusting environment with acceptance and support of mental health team allows the patients to develop a sense of power and self-control in a consistence, caring milieu.

KEY POINTS

- Psychogenic amnesia is most common type of dissociative disorder.
- Psychogenic amnesia may be localized, generalized, selective or continuous type.
- Hypnosis, abreaction and supportive therapy are the treatments of choice for psychogenic amnesia although a majority recovers spontaneously.
- In psychogenic fugue, patient may assume new identity which is incomplete in contrast to multiple personality disorder in which existence of two or more distinct personalities are present, each of which is dominant at a particular time.
- Since the symptoms occur in conversion disorders are to reduce the mental tension, the person often displays indifference towards the physical manifestation. This is called as '*la belle indifference*'.
- Defense mechanism used for conversion disorders are conversion, dissociation, denial and identification.
- Active listening, communication techniques, continuous encouragement and support are core of nursing process.
- Active listening and communication techniques encourage verbalization of feeling, conflicts and information regarding traumatic event that led to the dissociation states.
- The ultimate aim of nursing interventions is to assist the patient to develop personal insight and to achieve control over their anxiety.
- Providing a safe and trusting environment with acceptance and support of mental health team allows the patient to develop a sense of power and self control.

20 Alcohol and Other Psychoactive Substance Use Disorders

The human use and abuse of alcohol and other psychoactive substances has been around since the beginning of history. Today alcohol and other drug problems have reached epidemic proportion with incidence rising in adolescents and young adults. Psychoactive substances include all those agents which produce stimulant or depressive action on brain and prolonged use of these agents can cause dependence and can lead to different mental and behavioral problems.

A. **DEFINITIONS AND TERMS:**

1. **Addiction:** A state of periodic or chronic intoxication produced by repeated consumption of substance (Drug). This includes an overpowering desire (Compulsion) to continue taking the drug; a psychological dependence upon the effect of the drug and detrimental effect on both the individual and society.
2. **Habituation:** A condition resulting from the repeated consumption of a drug and include a desire (not compulsion) to continue taking the drug for sense of well being. (It denotes some degree of psychic dependence but absence of physical dependence).
3. **Dependence:** Dependence may be physical, psychological or both. Psychological dependence referred to as habituation, is characterized by continuous or intermittent craving for substance in order to avoid a dysphoric state. Physical dependence is characterized by a need to take the substance to prevent the occurrence of withdrawal.
4. **Abuse:** Refers to person's illicit use of substance.
5. **Misuse:** Refers to a physician's prescribing a drug in a medically unacceptable way.
6. **Psychoactive substance:** It is one, which when taken into the body can alter consciousness or state of mind.
7. **Tolerance:** Tolerance is defined as the need of markedly increased amounts of the substance to achieve the desired effect, that results from repeated use of a drug.
8. **Cross tolerance:** Tolerance that develops to one drug as a result of exposure to another drug.
9. **Withdrawal**: A cluster of symptoms often specific to the drug used, which develop on total or partial withdrawal to the drug, usually after repeated use.

B. **CHANGE IN TERMINOLOGY:**

WHO expert committee in 1952 and 1957 first gave the term drug addiction for such problem. But later it was realized that addiction is no longer a scientific term because this word has been used in so many ways like TV addiction, Money addiction, Lottery addiction etc. In 1964 WHO recommended substituting the term drug dependence. But later word 'Drug' was not found suitable because drug implies a manufactured chemical, whereas many of substances associated with abuse pattern are naturally occurring (e.g. opium) or not meant for human consumption (e.g. Airplane glue). Later a new modified term was introduced as psychoactive substance use disorder. But recently 'Psychoactive Substance' word was dropped because it risked limiting attention to those substances that have brain altering activity as a primary effect, but it does not include chemicals with brain altering properties that may be ingested either on purpose or by accidents. So current term of such problems is 'Substance Related Disorders (DSM IV).

Table 20.1: Classification of substance of abuse

1. **Alcohol**
2. **Opioids:**
   - Natural–codeine, morphine, opium.
   - Semi synthetic–Heroine, hydromorphone hydrochloride, Nalorphin, Oxycodone hydrochloride.
   - Synthetic–LAAM (Levo Alpha Acytyl Methadone). Levallorphan.
3. **Cannabis**
4. **Sedative and Anxiolytics:**
   - Anti anxiety tranquilizers–Benzodiazepines.
   - Barbiturates.
   - Non barbiturates–Bromide, Paraldehyde, Chloralhydrate.
5. **Hallucinogens:**
   - DOM (Dimethoxy Methamphetamine).
   - DMT (Di Methyl Triptymine).
   - LSD (Lysergic Acid Diethylamide).
   - Mescaline, Psilocin, Psilocybin.
6. **Stimulants (Sympathomimatic Substances)**
   - Ergot Alkaloids.
   - Primary stimulants–Amphetamine.
   - Cocaine.
7. **Volatile Inhalants**
   - Amyl nitrate.
   - Anesthetics like nitrous oxide, ether, chloroform.
   - Butyl nitrate.
   - Hydro Carbons—ccl4, Acetone, Benzene, Gasoline.

ALCOHOL

History of alcoholic beverages consumption is nearly as old as history of mankind itself. Evidence indicates that fermentation technology is available with even the primitive and isolated human tribes. Alcohol related disorders are most common substance related disorders.

Epidemiology

It is third major health problem after heart disease and cancer. Alcohol is responsible for about 50% of all homicides, 25% of all suicides and 50-75% of road side accidents. Alcohol reduces life expectancy by about 10 years.

Studies show that in the USA about 90% of young aged from 18 to 25 years , 92% of adults aged between 26 and 34 years and 87% of adults aged 35 years or above had used alcohol in their life time. The male female ratio is 2:1 to 3:1.

In India in 1999, the Ministry of Social Justice and Empowerment, Government of India (MSJE,GOI) and the United Nations International Drug Control Programme, Regional Office for South Asia (UNIDCP, ROSA) decided to undertake a large-scale National Household Survey (NHS) to obtain information on the extent, pattern and magnitude of substance abuse in the country. This shows following current prevalence rate of different substances:

Drug type	*NHS (current prevalence, %)*
Alcohol	21.4%
Cannabis	3.0%
Heroin	0.2%
Opium	0.4%
Other opiates	0.1%

Source: National Survey, 2004

Pharmacology and Metabolism

Primary active ingredient is ethyl alcohol (mono hydroxy derivative of aliphatic hydrocarbon). It is absorbed rapidly along entire gastrointestinal tract with duodenum and jejunum showing the most rapid rate of absorption. Nearly 50% quantity is absorbed in 15 minutes and absorption is complete in 1-2 hours. The absorption occurs by process of simple passive diffusion.

Metabolism

About 90% of absorbed alcohol is metabolized by the body mainly in the liver, remaining is excreted unchanged in sweat, urine and breath.

Type of Addiction

Number of researchers have attempted to divide alcohol dependence into subtypes. According to one classification dependence is of two types:

1. **Type-A Alcohol dependence**: Characterized by late onset, relatively mild dependence, few alcohol related problems and little psychopathology.
2. **Type-B Alcohol dependence:** Characterized by early onset, severe dependence, strong family history of dependence, frequent poly substance abuse and long history of alcohol treatment.

Another classification of type of dependence by Jellinek is on the basis of pattern of use:

1. **Alpha alcohol dependence:** It is characterized by use of excessive and inappropriate drinking, no loss of control and ability to abstain present.
2. **Beta alcohol dependence:** It is characterized by use of excessive and inappropriate drinking, with no clear physical or psychological dependence. Physical complications (cirrhosis, gastritis etc) are present due to poor nutrition.
3. **Gamma alcohol dependence:** It is thought to be common in US. Such persons are unable to stop drinking once they start. If the drinking ends as a result of ill health or lack of money, they are capable of abstaining for varying period of time.
4. **Delta alcohol dependence:** Most common in Europe. Here person drink a certain amount each day but is unaware of a lack of control. This disorder may not be discovered until person must stop drinking for some reason and he feels the symptoms of withdrawal.

Etiology

1. **Genetics:** Alcoholism runs in families. The children of alcoholics become alcoholic four times more often then children of non-alcoholic. Monozygotic twins had about twice the concordance rate than dizygotic twins.
2. **Childhood history:** The childhood history of conduct disorders, ADHD and Antisocial personality disorders increase the risk of alcoholism.
3. **Psychoanalytic theory:** According to this theory:
   - Alcohol alleviates anxiety and many persons use alcohol for this reason.
   - Person with harsh superego who are self punitive turn to alcohol as a way to diminish their unconscious stress.
   - Fixation at oral stage of development also predisposes the taking of alcohol by mouth to relieve frustration.
   - Certain alcoholic personalities are more prone to alcoholism which are characterized by shy, isolated, impatient, irritable and sexually repressed.
   - A few persons also use alcohol to increase sexual performance but it is a myth because alcohol increases desire but decreases performance.
4. **Cultural factor:**
   - Asians, conservative Protestants, Jews and Muslims use alcohol less frequently than liberal Protestants and Catholics.
   - Specific social settings like college dormitories and army bases also predispose to alcoholism.
5. **Biological factor:** Variety of neurotransmitters (Dopamine, Serotonin and GABA) have association with alcoholism but not yet established.
6. **Learning theory:** According to learning theory, all behaviors are maladaptive learned behaviors. Temporary reduction in fear and

conflict strengthen the drive to drink. Release of anxiety arising from first drinking experience is source of reinforcement in alcoholism.

COMPLICATIONS OF ALCOHOLISM

- Medical complication.
- Social complication.
- Neuro-Psychiatric complication.

Table 20.2: Medical and social complications of alcoholism

Medical complication: Include alcoholic liver diseases, alcoholic pancreatitis, gastritis, ulcers, malnutrition, alcoholic myopathies, iron deficiency anemia, hemolytic anemia, alcoholic polyneuropathy, cerebellar degeneration, delirium tremens, alcoholic dementia, alcoholic cardiomyopathies, act as carcinogens for number of cancers, alcohol induced asthma and non-infectious aspiration pneumonia, sexual dysfunctions, wernicke-korsakoff psychosis.
Social complication: Alcohol is associated with increased morbidity and mortality, increased rate of accidents, increased aggression and violence (criminal and public), decrease in work-efficiency, increased absenteeism, marital disharmony, tension in families, separation in marriage and marital violence.

NEUROPSYCHIATRIC COMPLICATIONS

- Due to excessive use.
- Due to withdrawal.
- Due to chronic use.

A. Due to Excessive Use

1. **Alcohol intoxication:** Characterized by behavioral manifestations which depend upon Blood Alcohol Level (BAL).
   - *Stage of Excitement (BAL 25-100 mg/dl):* Characterized by sense of well being, warmth, increase of self-confidence and lack of self-control. The subject may disclose secrets at this point. An excitement of sexual desire is evident at this stage but characterized by prolongation of intercourse with delayed or absent ejaculation. Attention and concentration impaired, learning and retention become faulty. Person also experiences motor incordination.
   - Stage of Incordination (BAL 100-200 mg/dl): Usually manifest with excitable, irritable, quarrelsome and self depreciating features. Nausea, vomiting, facial flushing and pulse acceleration are common. Coarse or fine motor movements affected and ataxia and speech disarticulations are common.
   - Stage of Coma (BAL more than 250 mg/dl): This stage is marked by a depression of most bodily functions. Staggering gait with inability to maintain posture observed. Finally stage of stupor or coma prevails, which is characterized by rapid pulse and breathing, cold body and constricted/dilated pupil.

   Other medical complications of intoxication include fall/accidents, subdural haematoma, and Telltale sign (facial haematomas particularly around eyes).
2. **Idiosyncratic alcohol intoxication:** Usually characterized by severe behavioral syndrome develop rapidly after the person consumes a small amount of alcohol that, in most people has minimal behavioral effects.

   This disorder displays impulsive, aggressive behavior with danger to self and others. Person also exhibits confusion, disorientation, illusions, transitory delusions and visual hallucinations. The cause is not well known, but history of brain damage, encephalitic or traumatic damage may predispose this reaction. The aim of treatment is to protect the patient and others. Physical restraint may be necessary, Injection Haloperidol or Lorazepam is useful to control aggression.

3. **Memory deficit (Black out):** This denotes a sense of amnesia for significant events that occur in a drinking episode. That phenomenon lasts for a few minutes to a few hours.

B. Due to Withdrawal

1. **Uncomplicated withdrawal:** It appears after cessation or reduction of heavy and perlonged alcohol use. It is characterized by:
   - Autonomic hyperactivity including sweating, facial flushing, increasing of pulse, increasing of BP and mydraisis.
   - Increased hand tremors.
   - Insomnia.
   - Nausea or vomiting.
   - Transientry visual, tactile or auditory hallucinations.
   - Psychomotor agitation and/or anxiety.

   Patient may develop grand mal seizures in later stage.

   These symptoms significantly impair the social, occupational or other functions.

   Treatment of uncomplicated alcohol withdrawal include:
   - Benzodiazepine (Orally or IV) Chlordiazepoxide, Lorazepam or Diazepam.
   - Symptomatic treatment as per requirement with proper care of nutrition.
   - withdrawal seizures: No need to use anti convulsants but a few prescribed carbamazepine 800mg/day.
2. **Complicated withdrawal (Delirium Tremens):** Delirium Tremens is most serious problem with high mortality (20%), which usually appears after 48-72 hrs. of stop drinking. Patient shows unpredictable behavior which causes danger to self and others. The main feature is clouding of consciousness with disorientation to time and place. The other features include autonomic hyperactivity with tachycardia, sweating, hypertension, perceptual distortions (usually visual and tactile), fluctuating level of psycho motor activity ranges from hyper excitability to lethargy.

   It usually appears in 30^s or 40^s of age group after 5-15 years of continuous heavy drinking. The course is short with recovery in 4-7 days.

Treatment

To prevent delirium tremens, start 25-50 mg of chlordiazepoxide every 2-4 hours, until patient seems to be out of danger.

Once DT appear: 50-100 mg chlordiazepoxide every 4 hourly. If oral medication is not possible, I.V. Diazepam can be given. Other measures are to keep the patient in seclusive, well lit room. A proper diet with high calories, high carbohydrate and multivitamins is essential.

C. Complications due to Chronic Use

1. **Wernicke's encephalopathy:** A set of acute symptoms develop due to thiamine deficiency. It is usually manifested by ataxia, opthamoplegia, nystagmus and confusion. This encephalopathy may clear spontaneously in few days to few weeks or may progress into Korsakoff's syndrome.

   Treatment: The cause of this is Thiamine deficiency. They respond rapidly to large doses of parenteral thiamine.
2. **Korsakoff's syndrome (Alcohol amnesic disorders):** A chronic condition with irreversible memory deficits. It usually follows an acute episode of Wernicke's Syndrome. The possible causes are focal lesion in mammillary body and wall of III and floor of IV ventricles. About 80% of patients with Wernick's Encephalopathy develop Korsakoff's Syndrome.

   Treatment: Thiamine for a period of 3-12 months is beneficial.
3. **Alcoholic dementia:** The essential feature includes dementia that persists three weeks

after cessation of prolonged alcohol use. All other causes of dementia should be ruled out.

4. **Fetal alcohol syndrome**: Seen in infants of alcoholic mother. Mental retardation, growth deficiencies, craniofacial and midline defects, cardiac defects are symptoms of fetal alcohol syndrome. The cause of damage seems to be result of exposure in utero to ethanol or its metabolites.

   Other complications due to chronic alcohol use are Alcoholic hallucinations and Alcohol induced psychotic disorders, which should be treated with Antianxiety and antipsychotic drugs.

TREATMENT OF ALCOHOL DEPENDENCE

Why Alcoholic Seeks Treatment

An alcoholic seeks treatment because of following reasons:

- Pressure from spouse or employer.
- Fear of fatal outcome.
- Non availability of alcohol.

Patients who are persuaded, encouraged into treatment by persons who are meaningful to them are more likely to remain in treatment and have a better prognosis. The treating doctor has to help the patient to develop motivation by repetitively explaining to him about the harmful consequences of alcoholism. A motivated patient shows a better outcome.

1. **Psychotherapy:** One of effective treatments. The therapists need to be active and supportive during the therapy and discuss patient's problems sympathetically. The specific focus of therapy should be on:
   - Situations in which patient drinks.
   - Motivational forces behind drinking.
   - Expected results of drinking.
   - Alternative ways of dealing with those situations.

   Involving an interested and cooperative spouse in conjoint therapy for a few sessions are highly effective.

2. **Medication**

   A. Disulfiram: When alcohol is ingested, it is metabolizing to first acetaldehyde, and then it is oxidized to acetate with help of enzyme "Aldehyde Dehydrogenase". Disulfiram competitively inhibits the enzyme Aldehyde Dehydrogenase, so that single drink is usually the cause of toxic reaction due to acetaldehyde accumulation in blood. Those who drink while taking Disulfiram experience Antabuse reaction with symptoms like flushing of face, tachycardia, hypotension, palpitation, feeling of heat in face, sclera, upper limbs and chest. Sometimes patient becomes severely hypotensive, pale, nauseated which may lead to shock, myocardial infraction, hypoxia or coma. This condition needs an immediate attention by health professionals. Other agents used for this purpose are Citrated Calcium Carbimide and Metronidazole.

   Psychotropics: The commonly used psychotropics are Antianxiety (benzodiazepines), Antidepressant (SSRIs) and Lithium.

3. **Behavior therapy:** Behavior Therapy teaches the patient the ways to reduce anxiety. In this therapy relaxation training, assertiveness training and self control skills are useful techniques. Therapists also use two types of Aversive techniques (a) Electrical (Electrical stimulation to induce pain) and (b) Chemical (By apomorphine, and emetine to induce vomiting).

4. **Social support groups:**

   1. Alcoholics Anonymous (AA) is a self-help group of alcoholics. This organization was started by Dr Bob (surgeon) and Bill (a

stockbroker) in 1935. Its members make a public admission of their alcoholism and abstinence is the rule. It has been found to be helpful for many alcoholics.

2. Al-Anon is a self help group of the spouses of alcoholics.

OPIOIDS

Word "Opioids" come from word "opium", the juice of the opium poppy. The name of Plant is "Papaver Somniferum". This contains approximately 20 alkaloids, including morphine.

Classification

It can be classified into 3 categories:

1. Natural–Codeine, Morphine, Opium, Papaverine.
2. Semi synthetic–Heroin, hydromorphone hyrdochloride, Oxycodone hydrochloride.
3. Synthetic–LAAM (Levo Alpha Acetyl Methadone), Meperidine, Methadone, Levorphenol, Pentazocine.

   Routes of Administration are:
   Intravenous–Heroin, Morphine, Methadone.
   Subcutaneous–Heroin, Mepridine.
   Nasal–Heroin, Cocaine.
   Oral–Methadone, Percodan.
   Smoke–Opium.

Epidemiology

This problem is a severe threat to integrity of many countries. Heroin is most widely abused opiate in United States. The lifetime prevalence of Heroin use in U.S is 1.5%. India is also facing this problem because of its location. India is between golden triangle (consists of Burma, Laos and Thailand) and golden crescent (consist of Iran, Afganistan and Pakistan).

The number of heroin addicts also increased several fold in last 10-15 years. Heroin addiction is common in metro cities and eastern part of the country (e.g. Nagaland, Mezoram, Manipur, Assam, Arunachal Pradesh etc). The use of natural opium is also common in western part of Rajasthan, Punjab, Haryana and a few other northern states. The association of transmission of HIV and intravenous heroine use is now recognized as a leading national health problem.

Tolerance and Dependence

After continuous exposure of opioids, the changes in number of opioid receptors occur and these receptors need the regular supply of opium for their functioning. As a result dependence occurs. When the drug is displaced from these receptors the withdrawal symptoms occur.

Tolerance to opioid develops rapidly and can be profound. The terminally ill cancer patient may need 200-300 mg/day morphine where as a dose of 60 mg can easily be fatal to an opiate naive.

High Risk Group

High risk groups as identified in a number of studies for heroin addiction are:

- Low socioeconomic group.
- Certain upper socioeconomic groups and professionals like doctors.
- Persons with history of other substance use like alcohol, cannabis etc.
- Single parents and divorced families.
- With history of Psychiatric illnesses like depression, anxiety and antisocial personality disorder.

Clinical Effects

The clinical effects of morphine may be used as the model for all opioids. The analgesic effects peak about 20 minutes after I.V. injection or 1 hour after S.C injection and lasts for 4 to 6 hours. The other manifestations are feeling of warmth, dryness of mouth, flushing of face particular nose, euphoria (usually described as orgasm) followed by sedation.

Morphine has direct effect on brain stem respiratory centre and causes respiratory depression. Overdose can cause death due to respiratory depression. Heroin is pharmacologically similar to morphine. It is also excellent analgesic and has euphoric actions about twice as potent as those of morphine.

Intoxication

Opioid intoxication occurs after recurrent use of an opioids and characterized by altered mood, psychomotor retardation, drowsiness, slurred speech and impaired memory or attention.

An overdose is life threatening and causes marked unresponsiveness, coma, slow respiration, hypothermia, hypotension, shock and bradycardia. Death is usually from respiratory depression.

Triade of opioid overdose includes coma, pin point pupil and respiratory depression.

Management

- Opioid overdose is a medical emergency in which patient's respiration is severely depressed and he may be comatose or in shock. Ensure open airways and vital signs should be maintained. Opioid antagonists block or antagonize the effects of opioids, preventing them from acting. The antagonists include Naloxone and naltrexone. Antagonist must be used carefully because they can precipitate a severe withdrawal reaction.

Withdrawal Syndrome

Withdrawal symptoms begins within 6-8 hours after the last dose, peaks during 2nd or 3rd day and subsides in next 7-10 days. However some symptoms may persist for six months or more. The general rule is that substances with shorter duration of action tend to produce shorter, more intense withdrawal syndromes and substances that have longer durations of action produced prolonged but milder withdrawal.

Table 20.3: Withdrawal Symptoms of opioids

Behavioral	*Physical*
Anxiety	Sweating
Craving for opioid	Fever
Insomnia	Rhinorrhea
Anorexia	Mydriasis
Agitation	Piloerection
Possible violence	Nausea and Vomiting
	Profuse diarrhea
	Muscles cramping
	Cardiovascular instability hypertension, tachycardia
	Abdominal cramping
	Muscle/Bone aches
	Temperature dysregulation Yawning

Treatment of Opioid Withdrawal

There are two methods of treatment:

1. **Detoxification:** This process includes abrupt discontinuation of opioids followed by symptomatic management of withdrawal symptoms.
2. **Substitution method:** In this synthetic opioids like methadone can be given orally and substitute for heroin. It is given to addicts in place of their usual drug of abuse and suppresses withdrawal symptoms. Methadone maintenance is continued until patient can be withdrawn from methadone, which is itself addicting.

   Levo-α-acetylmethadol (LAMM) and **Clonidine** are other agents in use.

Other Treatment

It includes symptomatic treatment of withdrawal symptoms, individual psychotherapy, behavior therapy, group therapy and family therapy.

Narcotic Anonymous

Narcotic Anonymous is a self-help group of opium addicts. It has been found to be helpful for many addicts. Abstinence is a rule, and in order to be admitted to such a community, the person requires a high level of motivation.

CANNABIS

It is a major class of drug derived from hemp plant. There are three type of plants:

1. Cannabis sativa: 18 feet long, thrived in cool damp climate.
2. Cannabis indica: 4-5 feet long, thrived in hot dry climate.
3. Cannabis ruderalis: 2-3 feet long found in Russia.

The active psychoactive substance is delta - 9 "Tetra Hydro Cannabionol" (THC). Different preparations are named according to portion of plant used (see Table 20.4).

Table 20.4: Different preparation of cannabis

Preparation	*Portion of content*	*THC content*
Bhang	• Dried leaves and flowering tops of cultivated plant	1%
Ganja	• Small leaves and brackets of inflorescence of selectively cultivated plants	1-2%
Charas	• Resin from the flowering top of cultivated plants	6-14%
Hashish	• Resin from the flowering top of cultivated plants	6-14%

In United States the term marijuana is used to refer to any part of the plant.

Tolerance and Physical Dependence

Formally it was held that tolerance to various effect of marijuana did not appear to develop. However, some evidence of development to tolerance within few days of constant use is now available.

Withdrawal symptoms after chronic use of cannabis are usually mild, begin within few hours after cessation of drug administration and last for 4-5 days.

Complications of Cannabis

a. **Cannabis intoxication:** The symptoms with milder form of intoxication include impairment of consciousness, distortion of time sense and euphoric dream like state. Immediately after inhalation the person experiences light headedness, dizziness, sense of floating on air and a ringing in ears. Apart from these symptoms there will be reddening of conjunctiva, photophobia, lacrimation and the user may also experience tremors, ataxia and twitching. The effects of intoxication peak within 30 minutes and last for 2-4 hours.

   Severe form of intoxication is characterized by fragmentation of thought process and often by hallucinations. Person also experiences wave of ecstasy, perplexity along with depersonalization and derealization. Hallucinatory experience may constitutes of flashes of light, vivid colors, geometric figures, human faces or pictures.

   Management of this condition include: Good general support and reassurance, passage of time in a room with no external stimuli and symptomatic treatment if necessary.

b. **Acute psychiatric disorders:** As a result of cannabis use acute psychiatric disorders may develops. Such states are usually short lasting and self limiting and may be in form of Reactive emotional state and Acute paranoid state. **In Reactive emotional state** patient develops acute anxiety or hysterical dissociation leading to fugue like state with subsequent amnesia for the event of episode. In **acute paranoid state** or schizophrenia like disturbance the patient has delusion and hallucination of persecutory content. Such disorders are self limiting and do not require any treatment except in a few.

c. **Chronic psychiatric disorders:** Two such disorders have been identified in chronic users:
   - **A motivational disorder** is associated with heavy chronic use of cannabis in adolescents or young adults. It is usually manifested with lethargy, reduced drive, loss of interest in areas that were pre-

viously valued and lack of initiative in any work.

- **Cannabis psychosis** is a specific entity recognized in India, Egypt and Nigeria. After a history of chronic use person develops psychotic symptoms. Such symptoms can be relieved by use of antipsychotics and prognosis is good.

PSYCHOSTIMULANTS

A class of drug popular among students because of its stimulant effect was used to augment "Crash Study Programmes".

Drugs involved are: Amphetamine (Benzedrine), Dextroamphetamine (Dexedrine), Methamphetamine (Methadrine "Speed"), and Phenmetrazine (Preludine).

Pharmacology

Amphetamine is packed in various salts and mixtures, examples are like Methamphetamine-Amphetamine mixture, with other drugs like amobarbital.

After oral administration amphetamine's effects generally appear with in 30 minutes. It metabolizes through various hepatic pathways and significantly unchanged amphetamine appear in urine.

Pattern of Use

- Such drugs are usually prescribed for narcolepsy, ADHD or other illness. In low doses the toxicity and dependence potential is rarely reported.
- Intermittent low dose use is often seen in truck drivers, students and other athletes to overcome fatigue or the need for sleep.
- Another pattern of use is to induce euphoria when very high doses are used especially through intravenous route. High dose users often combine these drugs with sedatives and opioids to modulate stimulant effect.

Tolerance and Dependence

Tolerance may develop to some of the central effects of amphetamine like euphoria, anorexia, hyperthermia and lethal actions, prompting the chronic user to increase the dose in an effect to continue to obtain desired effect. The tolerance also develops to the cardiovascular effects. The phenomenon of tolerance does not develop to toxic effect on the CNS and toxic psychosis may occur even after weeks or months of continuous use.

Withdrawal Syndrome

After a period of chronic use, abrupt discontinuation of amphetamine is followed by withdrawal syndromes characterized by dysphoria, fatigue, depression, desire to sleep or hypersomnia.

In some persons hyperphagia, fatigue and depression are typically present after initial period of sleep. Withdrawal syndrome may last from a few hours to few days.

Intoxication

Physical Effects

The toxic doses seriously affect Cardio-vascular system, which includes Intra cranial hemorrhage, cardiac arrhythmias, acute cardiac failure, destructive deterioration of arterioles and marked raised B.P. An associated hyperpyrexia may be reported.

Neuro-Psychiatric Effect

Neuro-psychiatric manifestations after toxic doses of amphetamine include anxiety, insomnia, bruxism , touching and picking of face. Acute consumption of amphetamine may lead to a classical picture **of Acute Paranoid Psychosis,** which is virtually indistinguishable from paranoid schizophrenia. Tactile hallucination of bugs and vermines crawling under the skin (Formication) though not typical of amphetamine, have been reported sporadically.

Treatment

Aim of treatment is reduction in CNS irritability and sympathetic nervous system over activity with control of psychotic symptoms.

COCAINE

An alkaloid derived from plant Erythroxylon coca. The cocaine was first isolated in 1860 and became first effective local anesthetic soon. Cocaine (also known as Crack) is a substance of abuse in West Europe, but not common in use in India. It can be administered through oral, parental (intravenous or subcutaneous), intranasal routes, or by free basing.

Pharmacology

Cocaine exerts its effect by dopamine reuptake blockers. Psychological dependence may occur after a single dose. The effect of drugs usually last from 30 minutes to an hour after intranasal or intravenous use.

Clinical Effects

Cocaine is a CNS stimulant and effects are similar to amphetamine like elation, euphoria, heightened self esteem and improved performance of mental and physical tasks.

Complications

A. **Cocaine intoxication:** Cocaine Intoxication is characterized by extreme agitation, irritability, impaired judgement, impulsive sexual behavior, increase of psychomotor activity and manic excitement. The physical signs include tachycardia, pupillary dilatation, hypertension, perspiration, nausea and vomiting. High doses can produce seizure and death from cardiac and respiratory arrest.

B. **Cocaine psychosis:** Picture is similar to amphetamine psychosis and usually characterized by ideas of references, paranoid ideation, increased libido and bizarre behavior. Delirium with disorientation may develop. Tactile or haptic hallucinations like bugs are crawling just beneath the skin (cocaine bugs) is typical of psychosis.
Nose may be inflamed, swollen or ulcerated with perforated septum. The free basing may damage the surface of lungs.

C. **Cocaine withdrawal:** After cessation of prolonged and heavy use of cocaine person develops withdrawal symptoms. Such withdrawals usually reach a peak in 2-4 days and characterized by fatigue, insomnia or hypersomnia and psychomotor agitation. Patient also experiences dysphoric mood, anhedonia, depression and suicidal ideas.

Treatment

For acute intoxication the treatment consists of administration of Oxygen with patients head down. The Diazepam intravenously can be used for Control of seizures. Antipsychotics and Antianxiety agents can be used for associated anxiety and psychosis.

For withdrawal state a symptomatic treatment for withdrawal states include symptomatic use of tricyclic antidepressants and Dopaminergic agonists (e.g. Bromocriptine, Amantadine) to reduce craving.

HALLUCINOGENS

Drugs Involved

1. Lysergic Acid Diethylamide (LSD)
2. Dimethoxy Methyl Amphetamine (DOM)
3. Dimethyl Tryptamine
4. Trimethoxy Amphetamine
5. Psilocybin
6. Phencyclidin (PCP)
7. Thiocyclidine
8. Ketamine.

LSD

The classic synthetic hallucinogen LSD was first synthesized by Albert Hoffman, a Swiss chemist in 1938, who later accidentally ingested some of the drug and experienced the first LSD-induced hallucinogenic episode. It is also known as LSD-25 (25th component in a series of experiments). It is most powerful hallucinogen and oral ingestion of 100 microgram being sufficient for a significant effect in man. After intake the symptoms develop within 10-45 minutes and are back to normal in several hours to 1-2 days.

Effect of Drug

1. **Psychological effect:** The psychological symptoms of LSD are characterized by marked perceptual distortions, illusion, hallucinations (Visual, Auditory or tactile), depersonalization (Distorted perception of self) and derealization (Distorted perception of environment) with clear sensorium. Patient usually remains euphoric and is aware of that what he is experiencing is because of drug.
2. **Physical symptoms:** It includes mydriasis, tachycardia, palpitation, tremors, blurred vision, in coordination, hyperthermia and hyperreflexia.

Behavioral Complications

1. **Flash back:** Occasionally patient re-experiences the drug induced experience of visual hallucinations weeks, months or even years after period of drug-use. The flashback is often triggered by emerging from a darkroom or by use of cannabis.
2. **Hallucinogens mood disorder:** Features of anxiety and depression may persist even after weeks/months of drug intake.
3. **Hallucinogens delusional disorder:** Delusions may persist for variable length of time.

PHENCYCLIDINE (PCP)

Introduced in medicine as a dissociative anesthetic agent, but was to soon attain disrepute because of wide spread reports of delirious state while emerging from anaesthesia. That's why it is now restricted to the veterinary use only. It is taken orally, smoked or intravenously and symptoms usually begin in 2-60 minutes.

Drug Effects

1. **Psychological effects:** The low doses (less than 5 mg) of Phencyclidine causes euphoria, grandiosity, feeling of emotional lability. Higher doses (more than 10 mg) produce anxiety, excitement, perceptual distortion and synesthesia to paranoid psychosis.
   Patient also develops rigidity like symptoms to catatonic picture and toxic doses can cause even death.
2. **Physical symptoms:** It includes tachycardia, hypertension, vertical and horizontal nystagmus, ataxia, dysarthria, myclonus and seizures. The symptoms usually clear in 3-6 hours. Other complications include PCP delirium and PCD Delusional disorder.

Treatment

The diagnosis is based on presence of PCP in urine. The overdose of PCP can be fatal. It can be managed by hospitalization and gastric lavage and use of Antianxiety, antipsychotics drugs.

NURSING MANAGEMENT OF SUBSTANCE ABUSE

Nursing Assessment

In nursing assessment the patient's motivation for treatment is crucial to the outcome. Some people who are frightened by the effects of the substance on their health or behavior while under the influence of the substance may present voluntarily for treatment, whereas others are exposed to treatment subsequent to social and family pressure. If the person enters the hospital for another medical reason and is a substance user, withdrawal may become an issue. The assessment process includes:

- Identifying the type of substance the person has been using.
- The amount and frequency of use.
- The method of administration, and the length of time the substance has been abused.

The nurse should also take note of any suicidal ideation or intent, along with the presence of any withdrawal symptoms. If the patient is an alcohol user, it is important to ask about amount consumed, how often the drinking occurs, and the time of the most recent drink. Remember that most substance abusers underreport the amount they ingest. If the patient is seeking relief from his problems with a sincere recognition of the drug problem, an expectation of success is more realistic. A description of current drug use is obtained, including how much, how often, when use began, any attempts to decrease or discontinue using the substance. This information is reported to the treating physician. It is also important to determine why the patient is seeking treatment. As the nurse interacts with the patient during this initial interview, a therapeutic trusting relationship can be established in which the patient is accepted and respected for who he or she is at the present time. Long-term recovery is often marked by periods of relapse, or the reoccurrence of substance using behavior after a significant period of abstinence. The nurse should refrain from judging the patient or referring to this as failure. The nurse acts as a role model to demonstrate more effective problem-solving and coping skills. A baseline physical and emotional nursing assessment is done to determine admission status and provide a baseline from which to determine progress towards expected outcomes.

Nursing Diagnosis

Once the assessment data have been collected, the nurse determines problems that are created as a result of the substance dependence and its effect on the person's ability to function in activities of daily living. Potential nursing diagnoses of different domains (biological, psychological and social) applicable to the patient with substance abuse or dependence are as follows:

1. **Biological domain**
   - Acute confusion
   - Altered nutrition
   - Self care deficit
   - Violence self-directed or directed to others
   - Disturbed sleep pattern.
2. **Psychological domain**
   - Anxiety
   - Ineffective individual coping
   - Altered thought processes
   - Disturbed sensory perception
   - Hopelessness
   - Low self-esteem.
3. **Social domain**
   - Communication impaired, verbal
   - Social isolation
   - Non-compliance
   - Powerlessness due
   - Knowledge deficit of drug effects and withdrawal process.

Expected Outcomes

During the acute withdrawal phase, the patient requires a complete physical and emotional support to return to a more stable state of health. Detoxification is usually complete in 7 to 10 days. Once detoxicated, patient may have sleeping and eating difficulties along with the varied levels of irritability and anxiety. The nurse should remember that the patient of substance use without the drug is a person whose mind and body crave for the drug.

During this stage of treatment the nursing **short-term goals** are:

- Promote safety and protection of the patient from committing violence or suicide.
- Stabilize vital signs and general physical state.
- Promote and maintain fluid and electrolyte balance.
- To help the patient to take adequate food intake to restore nutritional balance.
- Promote a restful sleep pattern with adequate hours of sleep.
- Decrease anxiety and promote relaxations.

Following the withdrawal state, efforts are directed to help the patient to live a full and productive life as a useful member of society without the use of the substance. Expected outcomes with **long-term goal** of continued sobriety and abstinence from drug use are:

- Identifies the drug as a problem.
- Must realize responsibility for own behavior and recognize the association between the substances and personal problems.
- Identifies changes in lifestyle that are necessary.
- Maintains general health.
- Help the patient to control his impulsive behavior.
- Identifies alternative coping mechanisms to use in response to stress instead of the substance.
- Demonstrates efforts at positive change with interdependence on others.
- Begins to develop or reestablish a support system with family, employer, non-substance-using friends.
- Identifies available social support systems.
- Continues to abstain from substance use.

Nursing Interventions

Nursing interventions during the acute withdrawal state are directed towards controlling the symptoms of withdrawal without over sedating the patient. Nurse should encourage the patient to take medicine as prescribed. Benzodiazepines are usually the drug of choice for alcohol detoxification, starting with a relatively large dose with daily reductions until withdrawal is complete. If patient is in state of acute intoxication, a chart should be maintained for vital signs and medical care.

Nursing interventions with aim of achieving expected out-comes for each nursing diagnosis during acute withdrawal state include:

For protection from injury:

- Remove hazardous articles and furnishings.
- Assess for hypoglycemia and electrolyte imbalance.
- Observe for respiratory depressions, arrhythmias and seizure activity
- Initiate and administer withdrawal sedation.

For maintenance of health:

- Provide high-protein, high-vitamins diet.
- Record daily intake and output
- Provide pleasant and positive mealtime environment.
- Encourage oral hygiene.
- Provide free access to alternative nutritious beverages.
- Offer bedtime snacks.
- Weigh daily.

For care of Neurological-Cardiovascular Compromise:

- Determine level of intoxication and withdrawal stage.
- Provide a quite and safe environment.
- Record vital signs every 2 hours during first 3 to 4 days of withdrawal.
- Monitor neurology signs every hour until stable, then as needed.

To support emotional needs:

- Effort should be made to bring down patient's anxiety, fear, and hopelessness.

- Approach patient in calm, reassuring, and nonjudgmental manner.
- Encourage expressions of feelings.
- Reinforce patient's value as a person.
- Listen actively.

To remove denial of illness and non-compliance:

- Educate the patient about illness and addiction process.
- Listen to patient's reasons for noncompliance.
- Discus importance of regular treatment plan.
- Help to identify alternatives to maladaptive coping strategies.

For effective individual coping and socialization:

- Initiate a therapeutic nurse-patient relationship.
- Encourage patient to talk about him or herself.
- Teach problem-solving skills
- Demonstrate appropriate role-modeling behaviors.
- Help patient to identify reasons for social isolation.
- Help patient to set realistic interactions goals.
- Encourage participations in all group activities.
- Refer to social services or community support services.

Evaluation

Evaluation process will depend on the anticipated outcome. A patient can be evaluated on following parameters.

- Patient tries to cope with withdrawal symptoms.
- When the patient no longer exhibits any sign or symptom of substance intoxication or withdrawal and maintains a level of orientation.
- Patient has not sustained injuries during the detoxification period.
- As the patient gains insight into the illness express a willingness to admit and take responsibility for his or her maladaptive behavior.
- Patient initiates socialization and feels secure.
- Patient sleeps well and takes food regularly.

As the patient gains insight into the illness, express a willingness to admit and take responsibility for his or her own substance problem, treatment process can become a meaningful step towards a positive recovery phase. Acceptance of this responsibility is the first step toward a drug-free existence.

KEY POINTS

- Dependence may be physical, psychological or both. Psychological dependence referred to as habituation, is characterized by continuous or intermittent craving for substance in order to avoid a dysphoric state. Physical dependence is characterized by a need to take the substance to prevent the occurrence of a withdrawal.
- The important pattern of substance use disorders include—Acute intoxication, Withdrawal state and Dependence disorder.
- When the blood alcohol concentration reaches 0.1% person is considered intoxicated.
- According to Jellineck there are five types of alcohol dependence:
  - Alpha alcoholism
  - Beta alcoholism
  - Gamma alcoholism
  - Delta alcoholism
  - Epsilon alcoholism.

- Blood alcohol level of more than 100 mg% is usually manifested with coarse and fine motor movements, ataxia and speech disarticulation and is considered intoxicated state.
- Fetal alcohol syndrome leads to growth retardation, small head mental retardation and behavior abnormalities.
- Black out is a dense amnesia for significant event that occur in a drinking episode. This phenomenon lasts for a few minutes to a few hours.
- Cannabis, cocaine and LSD does not produce physical dependence.
- Delirium tremens is most severe alcohol withdrawal syndrome which appear within 2-4 days of abstinence and recovery occurs within 4-7 days.
- The characteristic features of delirium tremens are clouding of consciousness, disorientation to time and place, hallucinations of visual and tactile type and reversal of sleep wake pattern.
- Chlordiazepoxide is a drug of choice which is being used for detoxification.
- Disulfiram is a deterrent agent which when taken produces Antabuse like effects in alcoholics due to increase level of acetaldehyde.
- Treatment of choice of acute Wernick's encephalopathy, Korsakoff's psychosis and initial stages of alcohol induced dementia in Thiamine.
- Substitution (or maintenance) treatment of opioid dependence consist of using methadone, LAAM and buprenorphine. For detoxification, naloxone, nalorphine or naltrexone are used. Carbamazepine and Clonidine have also been used.
- Synthetic Opioids like methadone can be given orally and substitutes for heroin. It is given to addicts in place of their usual drug of abuse and suppresses withdrawal symptoms. The usual dose is 20 to 80 mg per day (max. upto 120 mg per day).
- Recent intake of heroin (Smack) is clinically judged by pinpoint pupil.
- The triad of opioid overdose includes coma, pin point pupil and Respiratory depression.
- Depression is the commonest psychiatric disorder associated with drug dependence.
- India is between Golden crescent which (countries of illicit opium production) consists of Iran, Afghanistan and Pakistan whereas Golden triangle is formed by Burma, Laos and Thailand.
- Cannabis induced psychiatric disorders includes **Reactive emotional state** (acute anxiety or hysterical dissociation), **Acute paranoid state, Amotivational disorder, and Cannabis psychosis.**
- **Amotivational disorder** is associated with heavy chronic use of cannabis in adolescents or young adult and characterized by lethargy, reduced derive, loss of interest in areas that were previously valued and lack of initiative in any work.
- Tactile or haptic hallucinations e.g. bugs are crawling just beneath the skin (cocaine bugs), is typical of cocaine psychosis.
- Flash back (re-experience the drug induced experience of visual hallucinations weeks, months or even years after period of drug-use) phenomenon is typically seen in LSD and hallucinogen dependence.
- Accurate and comprehensive assessment is crucial in addiction treatment interventions. Evaluation should consider all substance for pattern of use, withdrawal symptoms and consequences of use. Comprehensive evaluation also includes investigating family and social support system.

- Denial of substance use disorders is the individuals attempt to avoid accepting its diagnosis and can be exhibited by attempt to rationalize the substance use, minimize the harmful effects and/or blame others.
- Nurse should use a non confrontational approach when dealing with patients in denial of their problem. Motivational interview approaches are most effective, using empathy and nonjudgemental approach and helping the patient to realize his problem.
- Several effective modalities e.g. social skill groups, psychoeducational groups, group therapy, and individual and family therapy are used in addiction treatment.

21

Personality Disorders

Personality disorders are deeply ingrained, persistent, inflexible and maladaptive patterns of behavior that are in conflict with a cultural norm. Because the behavior does not usually confirm to the expectation of society, it leads to the distress and impairment in all aspects of a person's life.

Personality disorder can be considered to lie somewhat in between major and minor psychiatric disorders. Due to better understanding of biological, psychosocial and psychodynamic aspects of psychiatric disorders and availability of structured diagnostic tools, personality disorders are more frequently diagnosed than earlier. Prevalence of personality disorder in society lies between 11 and 20%.

PERSONALITY

WHO lexicon of mental health defines personality as the ingrained pattern of thought, feeling and behavior characterizing an individual's unique lifestyle and mode of adaptation. It is the result of constitutional factor development and social experience. Personality is considered to be a dynamic process. From the structural point of view, personality has three components:

- I. Temperament : Biological component
- II. Character : Social and environmental component
- III. Intelligence : Correlates and controls overall expression of both components.

PERSONALITY DISORDERS

ICD-10 defines personality disorders as severe disturbance in the characteriological constitution and behavioral tendencies of the individual usually involving several areas of personality, significantly deviated from the accepted cultural norms. Disturbances of long standing duration, pervasive, usually start in early childhood or adolescence and continue in adulthood.

In DSM-IV personality disorder are diagnosed on Axis II. Axis I disorders are major psychotic disorder. All personality disorders are clubbed under three clusters. There are a few terminological differences between ICD-10 and DSM-IV.

Cluster A: It includes disorder in which patients have odd, eccentric and aloofness as presenting features. Personality disorders included under this cluster are paranoid, schizoid and schizotypal disorders.

Cluster B: Patients have got dramatization, impulsiveness and erratic ness as their core personality features. Disorders included are border line, (Emotional unstable in ICD-10) narcissistic, anti-social (Dissocial in ICD-10) and histrionic personality disorders.

Cluster C: Presenting features in this cluster is anxiousness and fearfulness. Disorders included are avoidant (Anxious in ICD-10) dependant and obsessive compulsive disorder. (Anankastic in ICD-10).

As per ICD-10, a patient with specific personality disorder must have the following:

ICD-10 DIAGNOSTIC CRITERIA FOR SPECIFIC PERSONALITY DISORDERS

A. There is evidence that the individual's characteristic and enduring patterns of inner experience and behavior as a whole deviate markedly from the culturally expected or accepted range (or norm). Such deviation must be manifest in more than one of the following areas:
   1. Cognition (i.e., ways of perceiving and interpreting things, people, and events; forming attitudes and images of self and others).
   2. Affectivity (range, intensity, and appropriateness of emotional arousal response).
   3. Control over impulses and gratification of needs.
   4. Manner of relating to others and of handling interpersonal situations.

B. The deviation must manifest itself pervasively as behavior that is inflexible, maladaptive, or otherwise dysfunctional across a broad range of personal and social situations (i.e. not being limited to one specific 'triggering" stimulus or situation).

C. The abnormal behavior pattern that is pervasive and clearly maladaptive to a broad range of personal and social situations.

D. There must be evidence that the deviation is stable and of long duration, having its onset in late childhood or adolescence.

E. The deviation that cannot be explained as a manifestation or consequence of other adult mental disorders, although episodic or chronic conditions of this classification may coexist with, or be superimposed upon, the deviation.

F. Organic brain disease, injury, or dysfunction must be excluded as the possible cause of the deviation. (If an organic causation is demonstrable, the personality and behavioral disorders due to brain disease, damage, and dysfunction category should be used).

1. Paranoid Personality Disorder

Clinical features: Patient shows features of suspicion and distrust. Similarly normal actions of others are misinterpreted in personal concern and considered harmful and threatening. Their suspicious nature leads them to be watchful, resentful and guarded in their interactions with others.

He may have tendency to bear grudges persistently, e.g., refusal to forgive insults, injuries or slights. Many a time they may have recurrent suspicions, without justifications, regarding sexual fidelity of spouse or sexual partner. Paranoid personality disorder is more prevalent in men and typical behaviors are often seen in early adulthood.

Co morbid disorders include other personality disorders (Schizoid, Narcissistic, Avoidant and Borderline personality disorder) and other psychiatric disorders like major depressive disorders, obsessive compulsive disorders, agoraphobia, and substance dependence.

2. Schizoid Personality Disorder

Patients with a schizoid personality disorder are withdrawn and secluded and demonstrate an emotional indifference toward social relationships.

Clinical features: These people are socially aloof and emotionally cold people and adjust poorly in society. These people usually drive fewer pleasures from things that are soothing and sensuous such as music, romance and beauty. They display emotional coldness, detachment or flattened affecivity and have limited capacity to express either warm, tender feelings or anger towards others. Sexual experiences are usually not desired. This disorder is somewhat more common in men than in women.

Co-morbidity: Personality disorders (paranoid, schizotypal and avoidant personality disorders), Axis I illnesses (Delusional disorders and schizophrenia).

Differential diagnosis: Schizophrenia, delusional disorders mood disorders.

3. Schizotypal Personality Disorder

Patients with these disorders exhibit strange and unusual pattern of thinking and communication. They often display a sort of magical thinking in which they propose to forecast the future of others or read the mind of others. Ideas of reference, perceptual disorders and illusions are common. They also experience increased fear and anxiety in social situations, which result in diminished ability to form interpersonal relationship. This disorder is usually apparent in childhood and adolescence. Comorbidity include other personality disorders (schizoid, paranoid, avoidant and dependent personality disorders) and Axis-I-disorders i.e. schizophrenia, delusional disorders. Differential diagnosis with Delusional disorder, schizophrenia and mood disorder with psychotic symptoms are important.

4. Borderline Personality Disorder

Persons with borderline personality disorder have a persistent pattern of unstable mood, self image and interpersonal relations. They have a marked tendency to act impulsively without considering the consequences, poor futuristic planning and marked tendency to become involved in intense and emotional relationship which leads to emotional crisis. Frequent suicidal gestures or attempts are also noted. Some patients have inability to delay the gratification of need.

Co morbidity: Involves other personality disorders, Axis I disorders e.g. substance dependence, major depressive disorders, post traumatic stress disorders. Differential diagnosis with other personality disorders, mood disorders, dysthymia and cyclothymiacs are important.

5. Histrionic Personality Disorder

A person with histrionic personality disorder displays a pattern of self-dramatization, theatricality, or exaggerated expression of emotions. Such individuals are easily influenced by others or by circumstances and have shallow and labile affectivity. They show inappropriate seductiveness in appearance or behavior and have over-concern with physical attractiveness.

These people always want to be the center of attraction. Excessive dramatization and excessive emotionality is depicted in their behavior, though interpersonal relations are shallow and unsatisfying. Histrionic personality disorder tends to occur more often in women but is also seen in men. Differential diagnosis from other personality disorders.

6. Anankastic Personality Disorder

This personality disorder is often referred to as obsessive-compulsive personality disorder. People with Anankastic personality disorder have preoccupation with details, rules, lists, order, organization, or schedule. They have excessive perfectionism that interferes with task completion or compromises with the efficacy and performance. Rigidity and difficulty in accepting any new idea or change are also seen in this type and these patients are usually of type A personality and suffer from physical complications of stress.

Major depressive disorder is the most common co-morbid disorder, others being OCD and anxiety disorder. Obsessive compulsive personality disorder is seen twice as often in men than in women. People with this disorder are often employed in situations such as research where precision and details are required. Differential diagnosis: OCD and other personality disorders.

7. Dissocial Personality Disorder

Clinical features: Those with dissocial personality disorder exhibit a persistent pattern of disregard of social norms, low tolerance for boredom, dysphoria, promiscuity, violence and early deaths. Person performs action impulsively and recklessly to avoid being sabotaged. Vandalism, fighting, explosive anger, the verbal assault are common. School expulsion, truancy and delinquency are among the problems in the person's history.

History of conduct disorder before age of fifteen, histrionic personality disorders, borderline personality disorders, substance dependence, impulse control disorders, major depression and anxiety disorders are common co-morbid conditions.

8. Anxious (Avoidant) Personality Disorder

A person with anxious (avoidant) personality disorder exhibits persistence anxiety, fear of being rejected socially, fear of being criticized and feeling of inadequacy. They have persistent and pervasive feelings of tension and apprehension and belief that one is socially inept, personally unappealing, or inferior to others. They often avoid social or occupational activities that involve significant interpersonal contact, because of fear of criticism, disapproval, or rejection. Avoidant personality disorder is equally frequent in men and women. In a person with this condition, the fear of new situation exhibits in childhood and tends to increase by adolescence.

Schizoid, dependent, border line and paranoid personality disorders, mood and anxiety spectrum disorders particularly social phobia are associated co-morbid conditions.

9. Dependent Personality Disorder

People with dependent personality disorder display interpersonal dependency, excessive need to be taken care and going to extremes to avoid abandonment. Often they encourage or allow others to make the most of one's important life decisions and have limited capacity to make everyday decisions without an excessive amount of advice and reassurance from others. This disorder is most frequently reported personality disorder in women. Age and cultural factors can contribute to the behavior. Children and adolescents who experience chronic physical illness or separation anxiety disorder have an increased risk of developing this disorder.

Histrionic, borderline and dependent personality disorders, mood disorders, anxiety disorders, and adjustment disorders are common co-morbid conditions with this disorder.

Differential diagnosis: Agoraphobia, mood disorders and panic disorders.

NURSING MANAGEMENT

Personality disorder as such is difficult to treat entity. A large part of problem is on deciding on treatment of individual personality disorders because of degree of overlap between the various personality disorders and other mental disorders. Co-morbidity and poor adherence to the treatment further add to the difficulties.

Combination of psychotherapies, individually tailored psychotherapy along with pharmacological agents has been used with variable success rates.

Following types of psychotherapies have been tried in personality disorders:

1. Psychoanalytic psychotherapy.
2. Cognitive analytic psychotherapy.
3. Cognitive behavior dialectic behavior therapy.
4. Milieu therapy.

Pharmacological agents are used according to the symptoms. They are not syndromal specific. Among psychopharmacological agents, antipsychotic and mood stabilizers are used for psychotic episodes and aggressive episodes in borderline personality disorder, schizoid personality disorder, paranoid personality disorder, and dissocial personality disorder.

Application of the Nursing Process

Nursing Assessment

Most often a patient is not admitted with a personality disorder as a primary cause for treatment. Treatment is usually desired by the family members or others as the maladaptive behavior of patient becomes problematic and disrupts the person's life. Substance abuse, depression, or suicidal acts etc are other psychiatric conditions which further deteriorates the condition and leads to admission. It is important that the nurse first develops a trusting relationship by using proper communication skills. Some assessment techniques that could be used are:

- Find out what events or behaviors led to the consultation or admission.
- Look for inconsistencies between what is said and what is observed in behavior.
- Note any resistance to questioning.
- Examine the level of anxiety and emotional status of patient during examination.
- Enquire about usual coping skills have patient used to deal with various stress in his life.
- Observe scars or cuts on body that may indicate self-mutilating behavior.
- Ask if suicidal thoughts have occurred and verify whether a plan has been made.
- Determine social habits and present or past relationship in which the person is involved.

Patients with personality disorders are often irritating and demanding, it is important for the nurse to recognize and deal with his or her own feelings. The patient with a personality disorder can be manipulative with nurses and other patients, so it is important to view the situation objectively.

Nursing Diagnosis

After a detail data collection through the nursing assessment process, a nursing diagnosis is made. Because of similar symptoms of many personality disorders, nursing diagnosis may be applicable for more than one personality disorder. These may include:

- Disturbed sleep pattern.
- Imbalance nutrition.
- Anxiety, related to unconscious conflicts.
- Ineffective individual coping, related to suspiciousness, ambivalence, or projection.
- Personal identity confusion, related to social withdrawal.
- Personal identity disturbance, related to splitting and unmet dependency needs.
- Impaired communication, related to social withdrawal.
- Impaired social interaction.
- Low self-esteem.
- Risk for self-mutilation.
- Ineffective therapeutic regimen management.
- Powerlessness, related to extreme feelings of dependency.

Expected Outcomes

Effectiveness of nursing interventions can be measured by expected outcome. Nurses and patients work together to facilitate change within a reasonable time. If the expected changes do not occur within the given timeframe, the nursing care plan is to be revised. Anticipated outcomes for a patient of personality disorder are:

- Refrain from harming self or others.
- Decrease manipulative behaviors.
- Gain control over impulses.
- Exhibit decreased hostility and anger.
- Express thoughts and feelings appropriately.
- Participate in unit activities.
- Claim ownership of own feelings and thoughts.
- Increase interaction with others.

- Verbalize positive qualities about self.
- Make independent decision about self-care.
- Manage anxiety without acting-out behaviors.

Nursing Interventions

Providing care to patients with personality disorder is a challenging one. The nurse must identify personal feelings about the patient's behaviors and be alert of patient's manipulative behavior. Nursing actions may include the following:

- Show acceptance of the person at all times by separating the person from the behaviors.
- Provide a safe environment, especially important for patients with self-mutilating behavior.
- Develop a no-harm contract with the patient with self-destructive tendencies.
- Communicate information about patient's risk to other mental health team members.
- Encourage the patient to openly express his feelings and thoughts.
- Explain all unit rules and enforce them fairly and consistently and encourage the patient to participate in unit activities.
- Discuss with the patient how his behavior affects others and assist him to explore alternative actions.
- Provide positive feedback to patients who are making effort to change behavior.
- Assist and educate the patient in the problem-solving process and encourage him to keep a private journal of thoughts and feelings.
- Group therapy helps patients to improve interaction skills in addition to gaining an understanding of how they are perceived by others. Patients can learn how to ventilate anxiety and trust others in a safe environment. Problem-solving methods can be practised within the group to resolve community issues.
- Occupational therapy allows patients to increase their level of functioning so that they become more independent.
- Recreation therapy can assist patients to ventilate feelings and increase socialization skills.

Evaluation

The chances of improvement are limited because of their deeply ingrained patterns of pervasive behaviors that they have developed over time. The effectiveness of interventions for patient with personality disorder is difficult to measure. Changes do not occur quickly. A short-term outcome that involves interaction with other patients and impulse control can be evaluated within the confined milieu. The patient's behavior following discharge will demonstrate whether actual improvement has occurred or not.

KEY POINTS

- **Personality** is the ingrained pattern of thought, feeling and behavior characterizing an individual's unique lifestyle and mode of adaptation. It is the result of constitutional factor development and social experience.
- **Personality disorders** as severe disturbances in the characteriological constitution and behavioral tendencies of the individual usually involving several areas of personality, significantly deviated from the accepted cultural norms. Disturbances should be of long standing duration, pervasive, usually start in early childhood or adolescence and continue in adulthood.
- DSM IV has identified three clusters named cluster A,B and C.
- Cluster-A personality disorders included are paranoid, schizoid and schizotypal disorders.

- Cluster-B personality disorders included are: borderline, narcissistic, anti-social and histrionic personality disorders.
- Cluster-C personality disorders included are: avoidant, dependant and obsessive compulsive disorder.
- Obsessive compulsive or anankastic personality is characterized by perfectionism, punctuality, liking cleanliness, parsimonious, disciplined, excessive devotion to work, restricted ability to express warm and tender relations, indecisiveness etc.
- Schizoid personality is characterized by emotional coldness, and aloofness, shy, introvert, indifference to praise or criticism, few friends etc.
- Histrionic personality is characterized by dramatic behavior, emotionally immature, manipulative, attention seeking, narcissistic, dependent, suggestible and seductive behavior.
- Treatment of choice of personality disorder is psychotherapy (individual or group).
- Anti-social personality is characterized by inability to tolerate frustration, disliking supervision, inability to learn from experience, failure to conform to social norms, impulsivity, disregard for truth, recklessness, impulsivity, proneness for criminal and antisocial activities.
- Providing care to patients with personality disorder is a challenging one. The nurse must identify personal feelings about the patient's behaviors and be alert of patient's manipulative behavior.
- The chances of improvement are limited because of their deeply ingrained patterns of pervasive behaviors that they have developed over time. The effectiveness of interventions for patient with personality disorder is difficult to measure.

22

Eating Disorders

Like all psychiatric disorders eating disorders e.g. anorexia nervosa and bulimia nervosa are also syndromes. They are a cluster of symptoms. With Indian culture becoming more permissive to western influences, these disorders are likely to rise in Indian sub-continent. Beauty contests and attractive modeling career options becoming available in glamour market and staying in shape and slim are in demand in adolescent females. Transcultural studies reveal that these disorders are on the rise when non-western countries are exposed to western ideals of thinness.

EPIDEMIOLOGY

Partial eating disorders are more common than going by strict diagnostic criteria. Average prevalence for anorexia nervosa is 0.28%. Bulimia nervosa prevalence ranges from 0.1% to 1%. Male to female ratio is very much in favor of females, 10-20 times higher than males.

ANOREXIA NERVOSA

Anorexia nervosa is a disorder characterized by deliberate weight loss induced and/or sustained by the patient. The disorder occurs most commonly in adolescent girls and young women, but at times also seen in adolescent boys and young men.

Fundamental etiology of it remains elusive. It is a cluster of symptoms which includes under nutrition of varying severity with secondary endocrine and metabolic changes and distúrbance of bodily function.

Specific causes for eating disorders are unknown. These disorders are understood as interplay of sociocultural, psychological and physical factors.

Clinical Features

It is characterized by marked weight loss, (at least 15% below the normal), amenorrhoea, poor psychosocial and sexual adjustments with preserved mind alertness and denial of illness. Two patterns of reduced caloric intake are observed. In one type patients consistently avoid or restrict all types of food. Special attention is paid towards restriction of carbohydrate and fat rich foods. In second variant patient engages in binge eating pattern followed by self induced vomiting and purging. Binge eating pattern seems familiar with bulimia but these patients had marked loss of weight and meet other criteria of anorexia nervosa. Intense fear of gaining weight and frequent mirror gazing is also seen. Perception of body weight and image are significantly distorted. Patients usually fail to recognize they are emaciated. Impaired release of gonadotropin releasing hormone (Gn RH) release leads to impaired release of follicle stimulating hormone (FSH) and leutinizing hormone (LH), which further leads to impaired ovarian function resulting in amenorrhoea.

Medical Complications

Due to weight loss: Temperature dysregulation, poor maintenance of core temperature, low metabolic rates, cachexia, poor contractility of cardiac muscles and arrhythmias, amenorrhoea, edema, leucopenia, poor gastric emptying and abnormal taste sensation due to zinc deficiency.

Differential Diagnosis

Anorexia nervosa should be differentiated from loss of appetite in depression. In depression, patient usually reports of anorexia, but in anorexia nervosa, there is a total denial of loss of appetite.

Course and Prognosis

Approximately 25% patients recover fully after the first episode, 50% patients improve markedly and function fairly well. Overall there is 7% mortality rate and rest of the patients recover poorly—physically as well as socially.

Treatment

For management of anorexic patients hospitalization with specialized nursing care is advisable rather than outpatient treatment. Nutritional management should be combined with psychological modes of treatment. Patients with recent onset of illness, with restrictive type of illness and good family support may be benefited from out patient treatment. Inpatient treatment includes: Nursing care, dietary management.

Nursing care: Supervision, empathy with patient, explaining about the illness along with establishment of good rapport are prerequisites for successful treatment. Each meal should be supervised. Meal should be served in groups of patients and finishing of food should be mandatory. Details of nursing management are given below.

Dietary management: Nutritional management should be started with 1400 calories per day for initial 5-7 days, thereafter it should be increased gradually. It has been found for each kilogram of weight gain, 7500 surplus calories are required.

Pharmacotherapy: Cyproheptadine has been helpful for increasing dietary intake. Other co-morbid psychiatric conditions unlike depression; border line personality disorder etc. should be treated as per their guidelines. Other non-pharmacotherapeutic measures are cognitive behavior therapy and family therapy.

BULIMIA NERVOSA

Bulimia Nervosa is a syndrome characterized by repeated bouts of overeating and an excessive preoccupation with control of body weight, leading the patient to adopt extreme measures, such as self-induced vomiting or purging by abuse of laxative, so as to counteract the fattening effect of ingested food.

Repeated vomiting is likely to give rise to disturbances of body electrolytes, physical complication (tetany, epileptic seizures, cardiac arrhythmias, muscular weakness and further severe loss of weight).

Etiology

Bulimia also occurs mostly in young females, but at a slightly higher age than anorexia nervosa. These two disorders are closely connected in many ways. Similar etiological factors and attitude towards weight and shape are found in both. In many, bulimia follows anorexia nervosa.

Clinical Features

Like anorexia nervosa, bulimic patients are also concerned about their body shape, image and body weight but they are not as motivated to lose weight as anorexia nervosa patients. It usually presents as periods of dieting interrupted by binge eating episodes. Episodes of binge eating usually last for one hour during which patient eats high calorie food and eats it very rapidly. The episode is terminated by abdominal discomfort or social interruption. Binging leads to self reproach or guilt which in turn results in manual or pharmacological self-induction of vomiting by using agents.

Impulsivity is also depicted in other spheres of life in bulimic patients, for example, substance abuse, impulsive stealing. They have chaotic life and poor psychosocial adjustments.

Medical Complications

Due to purging/vomiting, patients develop electrolyte disturbances (Hypokalemia, hypochloremia, hypomagnesemia), inflammation of salivary and pancreatic glands; esophageal, gastric and dental erosions, fatigue, seizures and cognitive impairment.

Course and Prognosis

About 50% of Bulimic patients show signs of full recovery on long term follow up. Among recovered about one third relapse within 4 years. Twenty per cent patients continue to remain ill and meet criteria of bulimia nervosa. Overall there is 0 to 3% mortality.

Treatment

Cognitive behavior therapy, family therapy and interpersonal therapy are non-pharmacological measures used for treatment for bulimia nervosa. Pharmacotherapy includes SSRI (Fluoxetine), TCA and monoamine oxidase inhibitors. In 20% cases treatment with any of the above medicines leads to cessation of binge eating and in 60% cases, it leads to reduction in episodes. Long term effect of these drugs needs to be evaluated.

OBESITY

Obesity may be associated with psychological factors in several ways. Distressing events like bereavement, accidents and other trauma leads to excessive eating and weight gain in some. Obesity may be a cause for psychological disturbances in many, because it makes an individual sensitive about his appearance and leads to lack of confidence in his interpersonal relationship.

Obesity caused by drugs, endocrinal factors or constitutional factors is not included here. Treatment depends upon the underlying cause. Psychotherapy with/or without antidepressants may be helpful.

ROLE OF NURSE

For patients of anorexia nervosa, the goal of treatment should be correction of the maladaptive patterns of eating and thinking about food, where as for patient of bulimia nervosa focus should be on to stop the behaviors of binging and purging, as normal eating patterns are restored. Cognitive-behavioral therapy addresses the psychologic issues of both disorders.

Family therapy focuses on modifying the family dynamics to allow recovery to occur. Inclusion of the family in the treatment plan and counseling sessions help the family members to see how the maladaptive behaviors of the family are associated with patient's eating behaviors. Gradual increase in caloric intake may also be used to help the patient to overcome fearful avoidance of food.

In patients of bulimia nervosa, psychotherapy helps the person take a self-inventory of eating, binging, and purging behaviors. Education is provided about healthy nutritional habits along with efforts to reorganize the maladaptive thinking related to food, body-image, and personal achievement.

Nursing Assessment

Patients with eating disorders mostly deny their problem and maintain their maladaptive eating patterns for several years before treatment is sought. Behaviors such as binging and purging by the person with bulimia nervosa are done in secret and may not be detected until more objective symptoms are noted. Nurse's approach is an important factor in gaining the confidence of the patient. The nurse must examine his or her own feelings about food, dieting, and body image to maintain an objective view of the patient situation.

A no confrontational and nonjudgmental approach of nurse is important to convey caring, willingness to understand and extend the patient's problem. Such patients are very sensitive to criticism, so it is best to avoid asking patient questions that can be misinterpreted. History of any insomnia or fatigue, increased feelings of intolerance to cold temperatures, change in urine output etc. are to be taken into consideration.

Nursing Diagnosis

The following are the nursing diagnosis encountered in the care of patients with eating disorders:

- Imbalance nutrition: Less than body requirements.
- Fluid volume deficit, related to vomiting, diarrhea, use of diuretic or laxative.
- Altered bowel elimination: constipation or diarrhea relative to laxative abuse and inadequate dietary intake.
- Disturbed sleep pattern.
- Anxiety.
- Disturbed body image.
- Disturbed thought process.
- Ineffective individual coping.
- Altered family process, related to family dynamics.
- Powerlessness.
- Social isolation, related to psychological barriers and concealing behaviors.

Expected Outcomes

Initial treatment should be focused on decreasing the patient's anxiety, stabilizing the weight loss pattern and normalizing eating patterns. Following outcomes can be expected during the process:

- Communicates his fear and anxiety related to weight gain and inability to maintain control.
- Consumes adequate nutritional intake to meet appropriate body requirements for height and age and maintain daily intake of 1,200 calories.
- Gains 1-2 kg.
- Communicates sequence of events or thoughts that precipitate anxiety.
- Ceases engaging in self-destructive behaviors (binge eating or purging).
- Participates in various activities appropriate for health maintenance.
- Verbalizes feelings related to changing body shape and weight.
- Express understanding of negative consequences of too little fat on body.
- Identifies positive aspects of her body and its ability to function.
- Identifies ways to maintain a healthy means of weight control.
- Identifies family roles and boundaries, and modifies them as indicated.
- Demonstrates improved interpersonal skills in social setting.

Nursing Interventions

The nurse has multiple roles while working with a patient who has an eating disorder. In addition to meet the physiological needs of the patient, the nurse may also function to provide psychotherapeutic interventions that include teaching, counseling, and being a group leader. Formulating a plan of care for the patient with an eating disorder should include the following actions:

- Weigh patient daily before breakfast by using same scale.
- Start behavior modification plan with privileges and restrictions based on food intake and weight gain.

- Maintain a strict daily intake and output record.
- Monitor status of skin and oral mucous membranes.
- Stay with patient during meals and at least an hour following food intake to monitor purging.
- Restrict time for meals to 30 minutes to reduce focus on food and eating.
- Convey to the patient that tube feeding may be employed if nutritional status deteriorates.
- Monitor amount and time of activity level.
- Regular monitoring of vital signs and electrolytes.
- Establish a trusting relationship conveying caring, concern, and commitment.
- Use a firm and supportive approach to eating and related behaviors.
- Clarify patient's views about ideal body by measurements and comparisons to norms for height and age.
- Assist patient in identifying positive physical characteristics.
- Encourage family to participate in education regarding connection between family process and the patient's disorder.
- Encourage participation in group and social role-play activities.

Evaluation

A number of factors influence the outcome of treatment for eating disorders. In anorexia nervosa, long duration of symptoms and low weight predict poor outcome, whereas family support and involvement generally improves outcome. Normal weight for height and age and normal laboratory values and vital signs, with absence of previous abnormal physical findings, will demonstrate a successful health status outcome. A regular follow up counseling and support toward continued abstinence from previous unhealthy behaviors is important in view of the high incidence of relapse.

Patients with bulimia nervosa have better recovery outcomes than anorexia nervosa. Experts report a recovery rate of 70% with cognitive behavior therapy and medications. Good outcome is associated with shorter duration of illness and receiving treatment in first few years of illness.

KEY POINTS

- Anorexia nervosa and Bulimia nervosa are predominantly seen in girls (10-20 times higher than males).
- Anorexia nervosa is a disorder characterized by deliberate weight loss induced and/or sustained by the patient, this disorder occurs most commonly in adolescent girls and young women.
- Weight loss should be at least 15% below the normal or expected weight for age and height in anorexia nervosa.
- Temperature dysregulation, poor maintenance of core temperature, low metabolic rates, cachexia, poor contractility of cardiac muscles and arrhythmias, amenorrhoea, edema, leucopenia, poor gastric emptying and abnormal taste sensation due to zinc deficiency are important medical complication of weight loss of anorexia nervosa.
- Nursing Care, Dietary Management and pharmacotherapy with cognitive behavior therapy and family therapy are important measures to be taken for management of anorexia nervosa.
- Supervision, empathy with patient, explaining about the illness along with establishment of good rapport are prerequisites of successful nursing treatment. Each meal should be supervised. Meal should be served in groups of patients and finishing of food should be mandatory.

- Bulimia Nervosa is a syndrome characterized by repeated bouts of overeating and an excessive preoccupation with control of body weight, leading the patient to adopt extreme measures, such as self induced vomiting or purging by abuse of laxative, so as to mitigate the fattening effect of ingested food.
- Repeated vomiting is likely to give rise to disturbances of body electrolytes, physical complication (tetany, epileptic seizures, cardiac arrhythmias, muscular weakness and further severe loss of weight).
- Electrolyte disturbances (hypokalemia, hypochloremia, hypomagnesemia), Inflammation of salivary and pancreatic glands, esophageal, gastric and dental erosions, fatigue, seizures and cognitive impairment are complications of self-induced vomiting; and self induced purging of bulimia nervosa.
- About 50% of bulimic patients show signs of full recovery on long term follow up.
- Cognitive behavior therapy, family therapy and interpersonal therapy are non-pharmacological measures used for treatment for bulimia nervosa.

23

Sexual Disorders

The threads of sexuality are woven densely into the fabric of human existence. Sexual behavior is diverse and it is determined by complex interaction of factors. It is enmeshed with one's personality and affected by interpersonal relationship, by life circumstances and by the culture in which one lives.

Rigid definitions of normal sexuality are difficult to draw and clinically impractical as sexual failure of varying severity is probably experienced by most people at some time in their life.

NORMAL SEXUAL RESPONSE CYCLE

Normal sexual response cycle consists of four stages.

Excitement Phase

This phase is brought on by psychological stimulation (Fantasy or presence of a love object), psychological stimulation (stroking or kissing), or a combination of the two. The excitement phase is characterized by vaginal lubrication in the women and penile erection in men. The parasympathetic nervous system activates the process of erection. The pelvic splanchnic nerves (S2, S3 and S4) stimulates the blood vessels of the area to dilate, causing the penis to erect. The nipples of both sexes become erect, although nipple erection is more common in woman than in men. The women's clitoris becomes hard and turgid and her labia minora becomes thicker as a result of venous engorgement. The excitement phase may last several minutes to several hours.

Plateau Phase

With continued stimulation, the men's testes increase in size fifty percent and elevate. The women's vaginal barrel shows a characteristic constriction along the outer third, known as orgasmic platform. The clitoris elevates and retracts behind the symphysis pubis. As the area is stimulated, however, traction on the labia minora and the prepuce occurs. Breast size in the women increases 25 percent. Continued engorgement of the penis and vagina produces specific color changes; these color changes are most marked in the labia minora, which become bright or deep red. Voluntary contraction of large muscle groups occurs, rates of heartbeats and respiration increase, and the blood pressure rises. The plateau stage lasts 30 seconds to several minutes.

Orgasmic Phase

A subjective sense of ejaculatory inevitability triggers the men's orgasm. The forceful emission of semen follows. The male orgasm is also associated with four to five rhythmic spasms of the prostate, seminal vesicles, vas deferens, and urethra. In the women, orgasm is characterized by three to fifteen involuntary contractions of the lower third of the vagina and by string of sustained contraction of the uterus. Both men and women have involuntary contractions of the internal and external anal sphincter. These and the other contractions during orgasm occur in intervals of 0.8 second. Other manifestations include voluntary and involuntary movements of the large muscle groups. Systolic blood pressure rises 20 mm, diastolic blood pressure rises 40 mm and the heart increases up to 160 beats per minute. Orgasm lasts from 3 to 15 seconds and is associated with a slight clouding of consciousness. The passage of fluid into the urethra provides the man with a sensation of impending climax called the stage of ejaculatory inevitability. Indeed, once the prostate contracts, ejaculation is inevitable. The ejaculate is propelled through the penis by urethral contraction. The ejaculate consists of about 1 teaspoon of fluid and contains about 120 million sperm cells.

Resolution Phase

Resolution consists of the disgorgement of blood from the genitalia (detumescence), which brings the body back to the resting state. If orgasm occurs, resolution is rapid; if it does not occur, resolution may take 2 to 6 hours and be associated with irritability and discomfort (resolution through orgasm is characterized by a subjective sense of well-being).

Refractory Period

After orgasm, men have refractory period that may last from several minutes to several hours; in that period they cannot be stimulated to further orgasm. The refractory period does not exist in women, who are capable of multiple and successive orgasms. Sexual response is a true psychophysiological experience.

CAUSES OF SEXUAL DYSFUNCTIONS

Causes of sexual dysfunctions are multiple but these are mostly of two categories:

1. Psychological.
2. Organic.

Psychological Causes

These causes are responsible for 60-80% of cases:

1. *Conflict:* (a) Relationship conflict (b) Internal conflict.
2. *Anxiety:* Worry about sexual act, performance anxiety.
3. *Personality and upbringing:*
   - Lack of affection.
   - Rigid or prohibitory behavior.
   - Avoidance of physical contact.
   - Insecurity.
4. *Ignorance:* Men equate their capacity for sexual activity with virility means manhood. Misconception regarding size of genital organs, hardness of erection, staying power in intercourse also generate anxiety and subsequently cause sexual dysfunction.
5. *Psychiatric conditions:* Like anxiety states, schizophrenia, depression, alcoholism etc. adversely affect sexual cycle.

Organic Causes

1. CNS: Multiple sclerosis, Spina bifida.
2. Diabetes.
3. Alcoholism.
4. Genetic Conditions like: Klinefelter's Syndrome, Turner's syndrome.
5. Miscellaneous conditions: Musculoskeletal disorder, cardiac and respiratory disorder, peripheral and vascular disorder, injury and operations.
6. Drugs:
   - Hormones.
   - Neuroleptics.
   - Antidepressants.
   - Benzodiazepines.
   - Hypotensive agents.
   - Anticholinergic drugs.

CLASSIFICATION OF SEXUAL DISORDERS

Sexual disorders can be classified according to stages of normal sexual response cycle.

A. Sexual Desire Disorder

It is characterized by persistent and recurrent avoidance of sexual intercourse with partner because of absence of desire for sexual activity (Hypoactive sexual desire disorder) or by an aversion to or active avoidance of sexual contact (Sexual Aversion Disorder). It is usually associated with strong negative attitude or feeling about sex.

This disorder is more common in females (known as frigidity) and associated with fear of pregnancy, unsatisfactory past sexual experiences and/or fatigue.

B. Female Arousal Disorder

This disorder is characterized by persistent and recurrent inability to attain or maintain the sexual activity. She will diagnose disorder if the sexual stimulation is not adequate in focus, intensity and duration. About 30-40% women report this disorder.

C. Male Erectile Disorder (Impotence)

This is to identify as difficulty in developing or maintaining an erection suitable for satisfactory intercourse. It is a common disorder with prevalence of 7-8%. About 35 percent males have occasional erectile dysfunctions. If erection occurs in certain situation like during masturbation, sleep or with different partners, then cause is psychogenic, otherwise we must rule out organic causes.

D. Female Orgasmic Disorder

It is called inability to attain orgasm which is reasonable for her age and sexual experience. It is a very common disorder, but underreported in clinical settings because of cultural factors. The fear of impregnation, rejection by sexual partner, religious orthodoxy and negative psychosocial influence are important psychological factors in causation.

E. Retarded Ejaculation

In this man achieves ejaculation during coitus with great difficulty. The causes may be interpersonal difficulties, ambivalent attitude towards plan of pregnancy, and/or loss of sexual attraction towards partner.

F. Premature Ejaculation

It is presented as inability to control ejaculation before the completion of satisfactory sexual intercourse. The diagnosis should be made when the man regularly ejaculates before or immediately after the insertion of penis into the vagina. It is mostly psychogenic in origin and common in those having more concern about partner's satisfaction.

G. Dyspareunia

It is recurrent or persistent genital pain occurring before, during or after sexual intercourse. It occurs in both male and female. The diagnosis should not be made when the organic basis of pain is found. This may result from tension and anxiety about sexual act that cause the women to involuntarily contract her muscles.

H. Vaginismus

It is an involuntary muscle spasm of muscle that surround the outer third of vagina, causing occlusion of vaginal opening thereby interfering with coitus. It mostly afflicts highly educated women. The cause may include sexual trauma such as rape, painful first coital experience or strict religious upbringing.

I. Excessive Sexual Desire

Both man and woman may complain of excessive sexual desire as a problem. The conditions include *Nymphomania* (for woman) and *Satyriasis* (for man).

MANAGEMENT OF SEXUAL DISORDERS

Various corrective therapies are now used to treat sexual dysfunctions. Before deciding on which type of therapy to use, a detailed evaluation whether or not the disorder has a psychological range is necessary. To rule out this, a complete medical evaluation including a medical history, physical examination and appropriate lab studies are necessary.

An assessment should involve:

- Focus on chief complaint.
- Determine which phase of sexual response cycle is affected.
- When the dysfunction did first become apparent.
- What are the situations involved.
- In erectile dysfunction, an impotence of acute onset is likely to be psychogenic where as insidiously developing impotence is more likely to be organic.
- Presence of morning erection, erection when coitus is not intended, nocturnal erection with masturbation rule out organic impotence.
- Premature ejaculation is always psychogenic.
- Detailed medical history and history of drug intake should be taken.
- History of local trauma and operation in genitals must be taken.

Treatment of Sexual Disorders

Treatment should be global with emphasis on intimacy and relationship, not just technique. Identify and treat psychosocial causes with dynamic psychotherapy, marital therapy, hypnotherapy and group therapy. Sedative may be temporarily helpful if anxiety is prominent. A good prognosis is associated with acute recent dysfunction in a psychologically healthy person with good past sexual functioning and strong sexual interacts. A new sex therapy by Master and Johnson with use of individual psychotherapy, couples therapy, sex education, behavior modification techniques and dual sex therapy with focus on decreasing patient or couple's anxiety about making love are effective methods of treatment. Recently sildenafil citrate and intra cavernosal injection of vasoactive substance have been reported to be useful in treatment of impotence.

SEXUAL DEVIATION (PARAPHILIA)

Here para means "deviation" and philia means "attraction", so we can say that it is deviated attraction. Normal sexual behavior is varied. It requires a biological substrate for psychological expression and is strongly influenced by socialization processes in which individuals learn the norm of their culture. When their sexual behavior become extremely divergent from the norm and when they are harmful to others, it is known as Paraphilias. These acts generally involve:

- Preferences for use of nonhuman object.
- Repetitive sexual activity with humans involving real or simulating suffering or humiliation.
- With non consenting partner.

Epidemiology

- Pedophilia is far more common than other perversions, 10-20 % of children have been molested by the age of 18 years.
- Onset usually prior to age 18 years, with peak occurrence between 15-25 years.

Etiology

Psychological: Person, who has failed to complete the normal development towards hetero sexual adjustment, usually develops deviant sexual behavior. A pathological attachment or improper identification with opposite gender partners also results in such behavior.

According to one theory a paraphilic examines his own or other's genitals to calm his anxiety about castration.

Organic causes: Though no apparent organic cause is detected, some abnormal findings are:

- 74 % had abnormal hormonal level.
- 24 % had hard and soft neurological signs.
- 24 % had chromosomal abnormalities.
- Few had seizures, abnormal EEG, and major psychiatric disorders.

Types

Paraphilias are specialized sexual fantasies and intense sexual urges and practices, which are repetitive in nature (at least for a period of 6 months) and distressing to the person.

Pedophilia

Most pedophilic patients involve sexual activity with a pre-pubescent child or children (age 13 years or younger). Patient must be at least 5 years older than child. 60% of victims are male and 95% of pedophilics are heterosexual. Most pedophilics know the child involved, usually neighbor or relative.

Exhibitionism

In such patients urges involve the exposure of their genitals to an unsuspected female. Orgasm is brought by masturbation during or after the events. Almost in all cases exhibitionists are male and need a shock reaction from female for satisfaction.

Transvestic Fetishism or Transvestism

It is marked by fantasized or actual dressing in female clothes for purpose of arousal and as an adjunct to masturbation or coitus. Some individuals with transvestism want to dress and live permanently as women.

Frotteurism

It is characterized by acts of touching or fondling a non-consenting person, usually in crowded place where escape is possible, particularly subways and buses.

Voyeurism

It is sexual arousal by watching unsuspected person who is naked or sexually active. Masturbation takes place concurrently.

Sexual Masochism

Arousal from being sexually bound, beaten or humiliated. According to Freud masochism is results from destructive fantasies turned against the self.

Sexual Sadism

Sexual excitement following inflicting psychological or physical harm on consenting or non-consenting partners. A rapist deserves this diagnosis.

Management

- It should be differentiable from the experimentation in which act is done for its novel effect.
- Disorders like schizophrenia, OBS may release perverse impulses.
- Prognosis is good if there is heterosexual coitus in addition to paraphilia, high motivation for change and is poor or in early age of onset, high frequency of act, no associated guilt and history of drug abuse or alcohol.

Treatment

1. Difficult to treat conditions, therapeutic alliance with patient is problematic because

of confidentially which poses major ethical and legal problems.

2. Paraphilics usually seek psychiatric care only after their paraphilic behavior comes to the notice of others. Psychotherapy helps the person to regain self esteem and improves interpersonal skills and finds acceptable method for sexual gratification. In behavior therapy pairing a noxious stimuli (electric shocks or bad odors) with paraphilic impulses disrupt the learned paraphilic pattern.

APPLICATION OF THE NURSING ASSESSMENT

Nursing Assessment

The nurse can play an important role in collecting information regarding problem related to sexual functioning. A nurse can assess the particular areas of problem and should ensure confidentiality and respect the private content of the issues being discussed. During interview a complete history of present sexual relationship (whether satisfying or not), nature of difficulties person experiencing in sexual performance, duration of current problem, history of negative sexual experiences if any, history of difficulty with sexual arousal, and history of discomfort during sexual intercourse must be taken. A complete assessment must consist of social and sexual history, psychosexual and psychologic testing, and physiologic studies of sexual arousal patterns.

Nursing Diagnoses

Common nursing diagnoses in patient with sexual disorders may include:

- Anxiety.
- Altered sexual functions.
- Low self-esteem.
- Altered, family processes.
- Role or identity disturbance.
- Ineffective coping.
- Social isolation.

Expected Outcomes

After establishing nursing diagnoses, realistic outcomes are to be set. Following outcomes are expected in a patient with sexual disorder:

- Understands and accepts his deviant sexual behaviors without feeling extreme guilt and shame.
- Refrains from deviant sexual behavior by conscious control of arousal and sexual impulses.
- Confront distorted sexual fantasies and thought processes.
- Develops more adaptive and effective coping and decision-making skills.
- Cooperates and participate in a treatment program to change behavior.
- Develops an awareness of the feelings and rights of other.
- Develops healthy interpersonal and sexual relationships.

Nursing Interventions

It has been observed in assessment that most of patients with deviant sexual behavior had some traumatic experiences in early sexual and emotional development. Cognitive-behavioral, psychodynamic, and trauma-based methods are important components of treatment program. Relapse is common during treatment of the paraphilic disorders. Willingness of the person to participate in a treatment program is an important factor in outcome. The nurse is integral to planning and implementing the treatment process. She must develop a therapeutic relationship with patient by using an empathetic and nonjudgmental attitude. Interventions may include:

- Encourage the patient to come out with his feelings and perception of the sexual problems.
- Ensure privacy and confidentiality during disclosure and treatment.
- Use communication techniques to guide patient to discuss self-esteem and guilt issues.
- Develop self-awareness regarding feelings about own sexuality and relationships.
- Encourage group and self-help activities.
- Collaborate with mental health team to facilitate behavioral change.
- Report any knowledge of sexual offenses or abuse to appropriate authorities.

Evaluation

Although most of the patients with sexual disorders do not come forward for treatment, it is essential for the person to develop an awareness of the problem and the stressors that contribute to the dysfunction.

Through an understanding of the consequences of the disorder, a person can identify and work to develop satisfying, acceptable sexual practices with alternative ways of dealing with sexual feelings. With a reduced level of anxiety and improved coping skills, the person is better equipped to communicate and interact in an appropriate manner.

KEY POINTS

- Normal sexual response cycle consists of four stages: Excitement phase, Plateau phase, Orgasmic phase and Resolution phase.
- Psychological causes responsible for sexual disorders are conflicts (relationship conflict and internal conflict), worry about sexual act, performance anxiety, lack of affection, ignorance, misconception regarding size of genital organs and hardness of erection. Such factors generate anxiety and subsequently cause sexual dysfunction.
- Psychiatric conditions like anxiety states, schizophrenia, depression, alcoholism etc. adversely affect sexual cycle.
- Organic causes responsible for sexual disorders are multiple sclerosis, spina bifida, diabetes, alcoholism, genetic conditions like Klinefelter's syndrome, Turner's syndrome, Drugs: like hormones, neuroleptics, antidepressants, benzodiazepines, hypotensive agents, anticholinergic drugs etc.
- Sildenafil citrate (selective inhibitor of phospho-diesterase type 5) and injectable vasoactive substances have been reported to be useful in differential diagnosis of organic causes and treatment of impotence.
- Dyspareunia is recurrent or persistent genital pain occurring before, during or after sexual intercourse occurs in both male and female.
- Vaginismus is an involuntary spasm of muscle that surrounds the outer third of vagina, causing occlusion of vaginal opening thereby interferes with coitus.
- Paraphilias are specialized sexual fantasies and intense sexual urges and practices, which are repetitive in nature (at least for a period of 6 months) and distressing to the person.

- The nurse can play an important role in collecting information regarding problems related to sexual functioning. A nurse can assess the particular areas of problem and should ensure confidentiality and respect the private content of the issues being discussed.
- During interview a complete history of present sexual relationship (whether satisfying or not), nature of difficulties person experiencing in sexual performance, duration of current problem, history of negative sexual experiences if any, history of difficulty with sexual arousal, and history of discomfort during sexual intercourse must be taken.
- Common nursing diagnoses in patient with sexual disorders are anxiety, altered sexual functions, low self-esteem, altered, family processes, ineffective coping, and social isolation.

24 Psychiatric Disorders Among Children and Adolescents

According to ICD-10 classification, psychiatric disorders with their onset in infancy and childhood or early adolescence can be discussed under the following heads:

A. Disorders of psychological development.
B. Emotional and behavioral disorders with onset in childhood or adolescence.

A. DISORDERS OF PSYCHOLOGICAL DEVELOPMENT

The disorders of psychological development are the disorders associated with developmental delay and which have their onset in infancy or childhood. Functions that are usually affected are speech, language, scholastic skills, biological maturation and motor coordination. Genetics as well as environmental factors are thought to play the role in the etiology, but in general the consensus is that etiology of these disorders is not known.

Discussing all the disorders of psychological development is beyond the scope of this book. Important ones will be discussed in detail and a brief description of a few is also added.

SPECIFIC DISORDERS OF SPEECH AND LANGUAGE (DYSPHASIA)

In these disorders, child does not acquire normal pattern of language, be it speech articulation, expressive or receptive language or any other aspect. Disorders cannot be attributed to neurological or speech mechanism abnormalities, sensory impairments, mental retardation or environmental factors. As a general rule, delay should be sufficiently severe to fall outside the level of two standard deviations. The language difficulty interferes with the child's performance in school and social functioning.

Specific Speech Articulation Disorders

It is a specific developmental disorder, in which the child's use of speech sound is below the appropriate level for his or her mental age, despite the normal level of language skill. For diagnosis, disorder should be severe enough to fall outside the normal variations for child's mental age.

Expressive Language Disorder

Specific disorder in which child's ability to use specific speech language is markedly below the normal level for his or her mental age. Generally, inability to produce single words at the age of 2 years and failure to generate simple two words at the age of 3 years is regarded abnormal. Receptive language as well as non-verbal language skills is usually within normal range.

Receptive Language Disorder

Child's understanding of language is definitely below the level considered normal for his or her mental age. They have difficulty in learning new words. In most cases, expressive language is markedly disturbed also.

SPECIFIC DEVELOPMENTAL DISORDER OF SCHOLASTIC SKILLS

Disorders in which scholastic skills are not acquired up to the normal level in spite of ample amount of opportunities to learn and normal mental age. Any other brain disorder or trauma should also be ruled out. These disorders are more common among boys rather than girls. Etiology is not known. For diagnosis, there is clinically a significant degree of impairment in the specified scholastic skill.

Specific Reading Disorder (Dyslexia)

This is characterized by specific and significant impairment in the development of reading skills. It is not accountable by any other reasons like mental age or decreased visual acquity problems. There should not be any lack of opportunities for learning in the form of inadequate schooling. All aspects that involve reading, reading comprehension skills, reading word recognition are affected. It is frequently associated with developmental disorders of speech and language. Academic failures, poor school attendance and problem with social adjustments are frequent complications. Errors of reading noted are omissions, substitutions, distortions or addition of words, slow reading rate, and words or letters reversal.

Specific Spelling Disorders

In specific spelling disorder main feature is specific and significant spelling impairments despite adequate reading skills. It is not accounted by low I.Q., poor visual acuity and inadequate schooling. Spelling errors are usually phonetically correct.

Specific Disorders of Arithmetic Skills (Dyscalculia)

Difficulties or impairment in specific arithmetic skills not explained by mental retardation or lack of opportunity for learning. Classical features are basic computational difficulties in addition, subtraction, multiplication and division rather than complex, mathematical skills like algebra.

PERVASIVE DEVELOPMENTAL DISORDERS

Pervasive developmental disorder is characterized by qualitative abnormalities in bilateral social interaction and communication and by stereo type and repetitive behavior. They are pervasive in all situations. Onset is usually in infancy and disorders fully manifest before 5 years of age. Usually there is no period of normal development. It is also known as **Kanner's syndrome**. All the disorders are more common in males except **Rett's syndrome**, which is exclusively seen in girls.

Childhood Autism

This condition was first described by Leo Kanner in 1943. Childhood autism is characterized by marked and sustained impairment in social interaction, deviance in communication and restricted or stereo type patterns of behavior and interests. Abnormalities in non verbal communications are present since infancy. It is 3-4 times more common in boys than girls.

Table 24.1: Signs and symptoms of autism

- Lack of reciprocal social interactions.
- Lack of responsiveness to others.
- Severe impairment in verbal and non-verbal communication.
- Repetitive behavior (mannerism, head banging, non-functional rituals).
- Unusual responses to environmental stimuli (erratic sleep patterns, pica, echopraxia and poor affection).

Etiology

As with other disorders of psychological origin, etiology is poorly understood. Twin studies show higher concordance in monozygotic twins and cognitive abnormalities in non-affected siblings. Fragile X syndrome and tuberous sclerosis are two disorders associated with autism.

Course and Prognosis

Most autistic children report poor outcome and condition remains stable with very little improvement.

Treatment

Education and behavior therapy are the main non pharmacological means. Skill should be broken into smaller fragment, so as to help the patient to learn each component separately. Care givers should be taught to help their patients repeat the activities learnt at the centre so as to help the generalization of the newly acquired skill.

Behavioral therapy is used for controlling disruptive and self injurious behavior. Positive reinforcement is used when the desired behavior is depicted. Antipsychotics are used for controlling repetitive behavior and agitation when behavioral models fail. SSRIs are used for controlling aggression and stereotypes.

B. EMOTIONAL AND BEHAVIORAL DISORDERS WITH ONSET IN CHILDHOOD AND ADOLESCENCE

Attention Deficit Hyperkinetic Disorders (ADHD)

This disorder is characterized by combination of over activity, poorly modulated behavior with marked inattention and lack of persistent task involvement. It is seen in 3 to 5% children in general population. Boys are 2-3 times more affected than girls. Generally, the disorder manifests before 7 years of age.

Etiology

It is seen to run in families. Monozygotic twins have concordance rate up to 80%. Siblings have 5 times more chances of likely to suffer than general population. In sporadic cases, problematic pregnancies, use of nicotine or alcohol during pregnancy, low birth weight and traumatic brain injury have been found to be associated with attention deficit disorders (ADD).

Clinical Features

There may be primary symptoms of inattention, hyperactivity, and impulsive actions. The behavior cause significant difficulty for children when adapting in home, school or social settings. The child with ADHD exhibits these behaviors with more frequency than any other child of the same mental age and developmental level and must have persisted for at least six months. Common signs and symptoms of ADHD are given in Table 24.2.

Table 24.2: Common signs and symptoms of ADHD

- Often fails to give close attention to details, or makes careless errors in school-work, work or other activities.
- Often appears not to listen to what is being said to him or her.
- Often fails to follow through instructions or to finish school work, chores or duties in the work place.
- Often avoids or strongly dislikes tasks such as home work, that requires sustained mental effort.
- Fidgety and frequent squirming with inability to remain seated when requested to do so.
- Is often unduly noisy in playing or has difficulty in engaging quietly in leisure activities.
- Often runs about or climbs excessively in situations in which it is inappropriate.
- Often blurts out answers before the questions have been completed.
- Often fails to wait in line or awaits turns in games or group situations.
- Often talks excessively without appropriate response to social constraints.
- Poor parent-child relationship.
- Poor peer relationship.
- Temper tantrum, low tolerance to frustration.

For making diagnosis of ADHD, report or history should be taken from various sources including parents, peers and school teachers. These children are generally poor academic achievers.

Subtypes

1. Inattentive type.
2. Hyperactive-impulsive type.
3. Combined type (most common type).

Course and Prognosis

Prognosis is not very good 60-80% of the children tend to suffer till their adolescence. Hyperactivity symptoms improve with age, but inattention symptoms tend to persist.

Treatment

Behavior therapy, training of parents, structuring of school activities, remodeling of class room behavior are non-pharmacological measures used in the treatment of ADHD. Positive as well as negative reinforcement should be used for promoting desirable behavior. Among pharmacological agents central nervous system stimulant are used for treatment.

Conduct Disorders

In this disorder of children and adolescence, person depicts persistent anti-social behavior. Dissociality is depicted in terms of cruelty towards animals and people, vindictiveness, cunningness, destructiveness and poor regard of social norms. It is supposed to be result of imbalance between protective forces and risk factors. Protective forces include good parenting, social support, proper schooling, and social ethics. Risk factors include poor personal performances, poor relations with the parents, poor adjustment in society etc. The role of inheritance is doubtful.

Clinical Features

Children with conduct disorder usually demonstrate repeated disruptive and aggressive behavior towards other people and animals. They willfully defy the family rules. Violations of age appropriate societal norms are common. Truancy from school, running away from home is common in school going children. In adolescent there may be an early onset of sexual promiscuity, substance use and physical violence.

Treatment

Behavioral Therapy, parental training, remodeling class room behavior are the main stay of treatment. Early diagnosis is helpful to start non-pharmacological measures at the earliest so as to avoid deterioration of psychopathology. Pharmacological agents are used for symptomatic treatment of anger out bursts, aggression and cruelty. Agents tried are SSRI, clonidine, beta blockers and antiepileptics.

TIC Disorders

Tics are sudden onset, purposeless, involuntary, rapid, recurrent and non-rhythmic motor movements of a circumscribed group of muscles or vocal productions. Tics are considered to be irresistible, but they should be differentiated from compulsions, as compulsions are done in a specific pattern and with a purpose. Both motor and vocal tics are differentiated into simple and complex types. Common simple motor tics are eye blinking, neck jerking, shoulder shrugging and facial grimacing. Common simple vocal tics include throat clearing, sniffing and hissing. Complex motor tics include jumping and hopping. Both complex vocal and complex motor tics are seen in *Gela de la tourette syndrome.*

Etiology

Etiology of tic disorder is not clear, though familial cases have been seen and abnormal dopamine levels are seen in frontal cortex, basal ganglia and thalamus.

Treatment

Psychoeducation should be provided to the patients regarding their illness and periods of exacerbation. Behavior therapy can be used. Tic suppression can be done by high potency psychopharmacological agents.

ELIMINATION DISORDERS

Enuresis

Involuntary or intentional voiding of urine into beds or clothes in a child of above 5 years of age is known as enuresis. It should not be due to any physical cause, for example epileptic fit or urinary tract infection. It is termed primary if the child has never been continent for the last one year. Secondary if the child has been continent for the last one year and developed enuresis. Usually the presentation is nocturnal but it can be diurnal when enuresis also occurs in day time.

Laboratory Examinations

Complete urine examination for ruling out any urinary tract infections and radiological investigations for tract abnormalities.

Course and Prognosis

Usually a self limiting disorder, most of the children achieve spontaneous remission after 7 years of age.

Treatment

Behavior therapy combined with psychological support is the mainstay of treatment. Regular voiding before going to bed, waking children in between and to make them to go to toilet by themselves and pass urine is a very simple, but effective behavioral mode. Bell and pad technique is used as promoting condition learning. A pad is placed under a child's sheet which is connected by a wire to a bell. If the child voids bell starts ringing waking the child. With time child learns to wake up before voiding. Pharmacotherapy can be used as an adjunct.

Encopresis

It is defined as repeated passage of feces at inappropriate places by a child whose mental as well as chronological age is above 4 years. It can be involuntary or intentionally. According to the presence of constipation, it has been differentiated into retentive type and non-retentive type. Like enuresis it has been differentiated into primary and secondary. In primary type, the individual has never achieved fecal continence. In secondary type, individual has been continent earlier.

Etiology

In retentive type, there is presence of hard stools in rectum due to constipation resulting in overflow incontinence. In non-retentive type, both psychological as well as physiological factors are involved.

Treatment

Education of parents about defecation process, reassurance and psychological support to the child and behavioral therapy are the main non-pharmacological measures used for treatment. In behavioral measures, timed interval defecation has been found to be successful. No pharmacological agents have been used with success in treatment of encopresis.

MENTAL RETARDATION

Mental Retardation, mental deficiency, mental subnormality and mental handicap are the terms used to refer to the same condition. The terms used in the past such as amentia, idiocy, feeble minded, moron, imbecile and oligophrenia had negative perceptions attached to it and have become obsolete.

Mental retardation is characterized by intellectual functioning that is significantly below average or an I.Q. of 70 or below. The onset is earlier than 18 years of age and is accompanied by significant sub-average intellectual functioning existing concurrently with related limitations in two or more of the following adaptive skills areas like: communication, health care, home living, social skills, community use self directions, health and safety, functional, academic work.

Classification

Classification of Mental Retardation can be based on its causes (Table 24.3), the psychological classification based on the level of intelligence (See Table 24.4) and the educational classification on the current level of functioning of the mentally retarded persons.

Predisposing Factors

1. Low socio-economic strata.
2. Low birth weight.
3. Advanced maternal age, increased chances of chromosomal disorders like Down's syndrome.
4. Consanguinity i.e. marriage among blood relatives leading to higher incidence of congenital abnormalities.

Prevalence

In the general population, 2-3 % of the children have an IQ below 70. Nearly 3/4th of such cases are mildly handicapped. About 4 per 1000 of the general population are more severely handicapped with an IQ below 50.

Characteristics of persons with various degrees of Mental Retardation are given in Table 24.5.

Table 24.3: Causes of mental retardation

Prenatal factors:
1. *Metabolic:*
   a. Aminoaciduria–Phenylketonuria, homocystinuria.
   b. Organic acidureas.
   c. Enzyme defects e.g. galactosemias.
   d. Storage disorders e.g. mucopolysaccharidosis.
   e. Lysosomal, peroxysomal disorders.
2. Neurodegenerative disorders.
3. *Chromosomal disorders:* Down's syndrome (most common), Fragile × syndrome (2nd most common), klinefelter's, trisomies, deletions.
4. Neuroectodermal dysplasias, tuberous sclerosis.
5. Devlopmental and migration defects, microcephaly, porencephaly, lissencephhety.
6. Cretinism.

Maternal factors:
1. Teratogens in the first trimester of pregnancy.
2. Intrauterine Infections e.g. TORCHES groups.
3. Placental insufficiency.
4. Toxemia of pregnancy.
5. Antepartum hemorrhage.
6. Radiation during pregnancy.

Natal factors:
1. Birth injuries.
2. Hypoxic Ischaemic encephalopathy.
3. Intracerebral hemorrhage.

Postnatal factors:
1. Infections of the central Nervous system.
2. Head injuries.
3. Cerebrovascular thrombosis of central vessels.
4. Post vaccineal encephalopathies.
5. Kernicterus.
6. Hypoglycemia.
7. Hypoxia.
8. Malnutrition, iron deficiency.
9. Child abuse.
10. Miscellaneous psychiatric syndromes–Autism, Rett syndrome.

Table 24.4: Classification of MR based on IQ obtained on Psychological tests

Mental retardation level	*IQ Range*	
Mild	50-70	educable
Moderate	35-49	trainable
Severe	20-34	custodial
Profound	below 20	

Table 24.5: Characteristics of person with various degrees of mental retardation

Severity level/ description	*Mild*	*Moderate*	*Severe*	*Profound*
Preschool 0-5 years	Can develop social and communication skills, minimal retardation in sensori-motor areas, often not distinguished from normal until late age	Can profit from training in social and occupational skills; unlikely to progress beyond 2nd grade level in academic subjects; may learn to travel alone in familiar places	Can talk or learn to communicate; can be trained in elemental health habits; profits from systematic habit training	Gross retardation; minimal capacity for functioning in sensori- motor areas; needs nursing care
School age 6-20 years training and education	Can learn academic skills upto approximately 6th grade level by late teens; can be guided toward social conformity	Can talk or learn to communicate; poor social awareness; fair motor development, profiles from training in self help; can be managed with moderate supervision	Poor motor development, speech minimal; generally unable to profit from training in self help; little or no communication skills	Some motor development present; may respond to minimal or limited training in self help
Adult 21 and over social and vocational adequacy	Can usually achieve social and vocational skills adequate to minimum self support but may need guidance and assistance when under unusual social or economic stress	May achieve self maintenance in unskilled or semiskilled work under sheltered conditions; needs supervision and guidance when under mild social or economic stress	May contribute partially to self maintenance under complete supervision; can develop self protection skillsto a minimal useful level in controlled environment	Some motor and speech development; may achieve very limited self care and need nursing care

Management

Primary Prevention

These steps aim at eliminating or reducing the conditions that lead to development of mental retardation. These includes:

- Education to increase the general public's knowledge and awareness of mental retardation.
- Legislation to provide optimal maternal and child health care.
- Prevention of heritable causes of mental retardation by family and genetic counselling.
- Vaccination during pregnancy against rubella.
- Precautionary use of medication during pregnancy.

Secondary Prevention

This aspect concerns treatment of the illness in order to shorten its course.

- Hereditary metabolic and endocrinopathies can be treated in early stages by dietary restriction and hormonal replacement.
- Emotional and behavioral problems of the mentally retarded children may be treated using appropriate antipsychotics, mood stabilizers.
- Comorbid psychiatric diagnoses are treated as and when required.

Tertiary prevention (Disability limitation)

- Parental counseling, teaching them how to deal with the child and how to bring out the best in him.
- Special education for the child which includes adaptive skills training, social skills training and vocational training.
- Rehabilitation of the child in suitable social and vocational environment.
- Institutionalization should be avoided as far as possible and should be reserved only for the profoundly retarded children.

APPLICATION OF THE NURSING PROCESS

Nursing Assessment

Mentally retarded child is usually referred for evaluation and management by parents, teachers, and other health care professionals. Parents are often frustrated with the child's inability to adapt to daily living. During assessment information is collected regarding the child, the family and related environmental factors.

Parents, teachers, and others social contacts of the child are usual sources of information regarding the child's troublesome behavior. A history should include the time at which the problematic behaviors began. The child's ability to communicate and interact with others is usually assessed and observed using play activities. Thorough assessment is also made of the child's feelings, self-image, distorted thinking, or other subjective symptoms such as abuse, depression, or suicidal ideation. It is important to assess communication and interaction patterns among family members. It is also important to determine the degree to which child's behavior and actions are disrupting the family functioning.

Nursing Diagnosis

Selection of the appropriate nursing diagnoses may vary according to the need of the individual child. Because the child is in a period of constant growth and development, assessment of nursing diagnosis becomes further difficult. Because many of these disorders may overlap and coexist in the same child, planning may identify multiple problem areas. Those problems that can be considered to all children and adolescents include:

1. Self-care deficit, (related to cognitive processing or maturity level).
2. Altered growth and development.
3. Personal identity disturbance (related to inability to recognize self as separate being).
4. Sleep pattern disturbance.
5. Risk for violence. (self-directed or directed at others).
6. Risk for injury.
7. Coping ineffective, individual.
8. Coping ineffective, family.
9. Impaired verbal communication.
10. Impaired social interaction (related to disruptive or inappropriate behaviors).
11. Noncompliance.

Expected Outcomes

Once appropriate nursing diagnoses have been selected, planning includes determining anticipated outcomes which the individual patient may be able to accomplish. Realistic time-frame will depend on the individual patient and the nature and extent of the problem. Expected outcomes may include the following:

For Children

- Demonstrates consistent progress in self-care development towards maximum potential and independence.
- Exhibits increased autonomy and reliance on self.
- Expresses positive feelings about self.
- Exhibits ability to control impulsivity and takes turns with others.
- Remains free of self-harm does not harm others.
- Participates in planning and implementation of behavior improvement program.
- Establishes effective alternative communication with staff and family.
- Applies improved alternative coping strategies.
- Verbalizes decreased anxiety during separation from parent or love figure.
- Identifies precipitating factors for anxiety.
- Chooses and initiates appropriate social interactions with peers.

For Parents

- Identify strengths and weakness of the child.
- Participate in planning and implementation of behavior improvement programme.
- Provides reinforcement of child's positive behaviors.
- Develops appropriate ways to cope with anger and feelings toward the child.
- Expresses feelings of frustration regarding child's inappropriate behaviors.

Nursing Intervention

Implications for nursing care of the child with a mental illness vary with individual needs of the child. Interventions may overlap in the child with more than one diagnosis. General nursing approaches may include:

- Maintain a safe physical environment.
- Identify capabilities of the child related to self-care.
- Provide encouragement to the child towards independent self-care.
- Establish a consistent pattern of reward for positive behavior and aversive stimuli response for negative behavior.
- Establish a trusting relationship by first using eye-contact reinforced with a smile.
- Use positive reinforcement for child's attempts at interaction with others.
- Provide familiar security objects such as a favorite toy, pillow, or blanket.
- Provide adequate supervision and limits for the child's activity.
- Keep sharp or hazardous items out of reach or in a locked area.
- Intervene to prevent injury from aggression or acting-out behaviors.
- Redirect and channel aggressive behavior into a controlled activity.
- Use headgear such as a helmet or hand coverings to prevent self-inflicted injury during behavior such as head-banging, scratching, or hair pulling.
- Identify any suicide risk, ideation, or action.
- Attempt to determine precipitating factors that lead to agitated and self-injurious behavior.
- Plan activities that provide a chance for the child to succeed.
- Provide a distraction-free environment for task-oriented activity.
- Identify association between nonverbal communication patterns and the child's individual needs.
- Include parents in discussion regarding events that trigger overwhelming fears and somatic symptoms in the child.

Evaluation

Criteria for evaluating the desired outcomes in the child will depend on the problematic behavior of child. It is anticipated that children with developmental disorders will increase their ability to interact and communicate with others. This can be measured by progress in their ability to trust others and initiate social contact with other persons.

Evaluation of the child with attention deficit or hyperactivity will include a consistent decrease in disruptive and dangerous behaviors along with the ability to function in a social or structured learning environment. Goals for the child with a conduct disorder are centered on the development of self-control and a decrease in impulsive behaviors. The outcome is measured by improvement in the ability to have satisfying relationship with both peer and family groups. Positive steps in developing self-esteem and feelings of self-worth should also be noted.

Interactions between the child and family with emphasis on whether they are coping effectively with the child's behavioral symptoms should also be noted. A positive outcome is demonstrated in the child's ability to function and adapt appropriately to the environment around him.

KEY POINTS

- Childhood autism is characterized by marked and sustained impairment in social interaction, deviance in language and non-verbal communication and restricted or stereo type patterns of behavior and interests.
- In specific developmental disorders of scholastic skills, child does not acquire the scholastic skills up to the normal level in spite of ample amount of opportunities to learn and normal mental age.
- Specific reading disorders is the most common learning disability in children.
- Conduct disorder is characterized by a persistent and significant pattern of conduct in which rights of others are violated or rules of society are not followed.
- Boys are more prone to conduct disorders, girls are more prone to emotional disorders.
- Pica is the repeated ingestion of nonnutritive substances such as dirt, clay, plaster and paper.
- Behaviour therapy combined with psychological support is the main stay of treatment in enuresis.
- Attention deficit hyperactivity disorder (ADHD) is a common disorder (3% of school children) characterized by poor attention span, distractibility, hyperactivity and impulsivity. Males are 6-8 times more often affected.
- Mental retardation is characterized by intellectual functioning that is significantly below average or an I.Q. of 70 or below. The onset is earlier than 18 years of age and is accompanied by significant sub-average intellectual functioning existing concurrently with related limitations in two or more of the following adaptive skill areas like: communication, health care, home living, social skills, community use self directions, health and safety, functional, academic work.
- Prevalence of mental retardation is estimated to be 1 % of all children.
- Mental retardation is defined as an I.Q. below 70.
- Type of mental retardation are mild (I.Q. between 50-70), moderate (I.Q. between 35-50), severe (I.Q. between 20-35) and profound (I.Q. below 20).
- Among mental retardation (MR)- 85% have mild retardation, 10% have moderate retardation, 3-4% have severe retardation and 1% have profound retardation.
- Down syndrome is the most common identified cause of severe Mental Retardation.
- In nursing assessment parents, teachers, and others social contacts of the child are usual sources of information regarding the child's troublesome behavior.
- Nursing interventions for the child with a mental illness vary with individual needs of the child.
- Providing safe physical environment, encouragement for independent self, reward for positive behavior and establishing trusting relationship are important intervention needed in nursing care.

25

Treatment Modalities in Psychiatry and Role of Nursing

A. PSYCHO PHARMACOLOGY

The advent of the modern era of psychopharmacology in the last half century represents one of the most significant milestones in the history of psychiatry. As more and more effective psychotropic medications came in, a greater number of severely disturbed patients were moved from confined settings to community living. The field of psychopharmacology has furthermore, contributed towards the development of psychosocial rehabilitation programmes and the reshaping of mental healthcare delivery system.

Pharmacological agents used to treat psychiatric disorders are called psychotropic drugs. Psychotropic drugs are medication, which act especially to modify the behavior, thinking, mood and higher mental function. These psychotropic drugs can be classified as follows:

1. Antipsychotic
2. Antidepressant
3. Antianxiety
4. Mood stabilizer
5. Miscellaneous.

It is important to understand the basic mechanism and adverse effects of all the drugs. With the advancement in the understanding of neurochemistry, the drug therapies are capturing the central place in the treatment of various psychiatric disorders.

ANTIPSYCHOTIC DRUGS

Antipsychotic drugs are also called "major tranquilizers" because of their calming effect, and called "Neuroleptics" because of their parkinsonian and other neurological side effects. They are divided into Typical and Atypical antipsychotic drugs.

Typical (Conventional) Antipsychotics

- Phenothiazines (Chlorpromazine, Thioridazine, Trifluperazine, Fluphenazine etc.).
- Butyrophenones (Haloperidol, Trifluperidol),
- Thioxanthenes (Thiothixene, Zuclopenthixol, Flupenthixol).
- Diphenyl butyl piperidines (Pimozide, Penfluridol).
- Benzamide (Sulpiride).

Mechanism of Action

These drugs act by blocking dopaminergic receptors. The blockade of D_2 receptors in the mesolimbic pathway leads to the therapeutic effects. The drugs also block other dopamine pathways, resulting in the various side effects. The blockade of mesolimbic pathway results in negative and cognitive symptoms, and the blockade of nigrostriatal pathway leads to the extra pyramidal side effects, and blockade of the tuberoinfundibular pathway leads to elevated prolactin resulting in galactorrhea and amenorrhoea.

These drugs also block noradrenergic receptors causing sedation and postural hypotension and cholinergic receptors leading to anticholinergic effects.

Depot Preparations

Depot preparations are given to those who are not compliant with daily oral medication. These preparations (e.g., Fluphenazine decanoate, Flupenthixol decanoate, haloperidol decanoate) are esters of the antipsychotic drugs, usually in an oily medium. Usually the effect lasts for 2-4 weeks after a single intramuscular dose. Side effects are similar to that of oral antipsychotic drugs.

Side Effects

1. *Acute dystonia:* Acute dystonia occurs in about 10% of the patients soon after the treatment begins. The clinical features include spasmodic troticollis, tongue protrusion, grimacing, spasm of ocular muscles and opisthotonos posture. The term oculogyric crisis is sometimes used to denote the combination of ocular muscle spasm and opisthotonos.
2. *Akathisia:* This is an unpleasant feeling of subjective restlessness leading to inability to keep still. It starts usually in the first two weeks of treatment but can continue through entire treatment.
3. *Parkinsonian effects:* Parkinsonian effects are the most frequent of the extra pyramidal side effects and occur in about 15% of patients. The symptoms often take a few weeks to appear which include: Akinesia, expressionless face, lack of associated movements, stooped posture, rigidity of muscles, coarse tremor and festinant gait.
   Parkinsonian symptoms can be treated with antiparkinsonian drugs such as the anticholinergic agents. However, it is important to evaluate at regular intervals as to whether the antiparkinsonian drug is still required since these compounds may increase the risk of tardive dyskinesia
4. *Tardive dyskinesia:* Tardive dyskinesia is a late complication of antipsychotic treatment, and occurs in about 10-15% of patients on long-term treatment. The clinical features are: chewing and sucking movements, grimacing and choreo athetoid movements. As the condition responds poorly to treatment, prevention is important.
5. *Neuroleptic malignant syndrome:* Neuroleptic malignant syndrome is an uncommon but dangerous toxic syndrome associated with high potency antipsychotic medication. It is characterized by symptoms of fluctuating level of consciousness, hyperthermia, muscular rigidity and autonomic disturbance. These symptoms are hyperpyrexia, unstable blood pressure, tachycardia, excessive sweating, salivation and urinary incontinence.
   It occurs usually with in first 10 days of treatment. The mortality rate may be as high as 20 percent. It usually occurs within the first few days of starting antipsychotic therapy or by increasing the dose. Incidence ranges from1-10 in 10,000 instances of antipsychotic treatment. Management consists of immediate supportive measures and stopping the antipsychotic medication.

Atypical Antipsychotic Drugs

Atypical drugs bind to dopamine D_2/D_4, 5-HT_2, alpha adrenergic and muscarinic receptors and therefore less likely to cause movement disorders and hyperprolactinaemia than the typical antipsychotics. Atypical antipsychotics control positive symptoms just as typical antipsychotics but also have a major impact on reduction of negative symptoms of psychosis. A few commonly used atypical antipsychotics are as follows:

Clozapine

It was the first atypical drug to be marketed. It is a serotonin 2A-receptor and Dopamine-2A receptor antagonist. It is particularly effective in the treatment of resistant cases. Clozapine does not cause extra pyramidal side effects, but it causes neutropenia in 2-3% of patients which progresses to agranulocytosis in 0.3% of patients. With regular blood tests and monitoring the cell count, leucopenia can be detected early. Once the drug is stopped, the white cell count usually returns to normal. Clozapine may also cause excessive salivation, postural hypotension, weight gain, hyperthermia, and seizures. Clozapine is sedating and respiratory depression can occur, especially in combination with benzodiazepines. Doses range is 200-450 mg per day.

Risperidone

It is atypical at lower doses but may cause EPS in higher doses. Risperidone is effective for both positive and negative symptoms. It may also improve mood in psychotic disorders, behavioral disturbances and cognitive functioning in dementia.

Olanzapine

It has a chemical structure more like clozapine. It does not cause EPS even at higher doses, but has other side effects, especially weight gain because of the antihistamine and serotonin $_2$ antagonist properties. Olanzapine also improves mood in schizophrenia and bipolar patients and may improve cognitive functioning.

Ziprasidone

It does not cause weight gain as it has no antihistaminic effects.

Other atypical antipsychotic drug: Loxapine, Sertindole, and Aripiprazole.

Contraindications

Important contraindications are hypersensitivity, coma or severe depression; liver, renal, or cardiac insufficiency; blood dyscrasis; and Parkinson's diseases. They are used with caution in older patients; those with diabetes mellitus, chronic pulmonary disease, or prostatic hypertrophy; and during pregnancy and lactation.

ROLE OF NURSE

The role of the nurse is significant when planning care for psychiatric patient, who is on antipsychotic drugs. An early observation and prevention of complications are important factors in mental health nursing care. It is important to include following nursing interventions for patients on psychotropic drugs:

- Nurse must be well versed with the accurate route of medication.
- Monitor expected reduction in aggressive and hyperactive behavior.
- Always look for possible side effects of drugs.
- Most of antipsychotics causes drowsiness. Medicine should be administered at bed time. The patient should be advised not to drive and handle heavy machinery while taking antipsychotic.
- Nurse should be well versed with extrapyramidal side effects of antipsychotic drugs. Nurse should monitor the patient for extrapyramidal side effects. An early observation, reporting and use of anti parkinsonian drugs can reduce the side effects of these medicines.
- Many of antipsychotics cause orthostatic hypotension. If blood pressure drops by 20 to 30 mm of Hg, immediate reporting and intervention is required.
- Most of antipsychotics cause weight gain so regular weight record should be maintained. The patient should be advised for low salt and low caloric diet.
- Patient should be advised not to alter or withdraw medicines without discussing with treating doctor. The drug should be withdrawn only under supervision of doctor.

Table 25.1: Antipsychotic drugs

Class and Name of drug	*Oral dose Mg/day*	*Parental dose*	*Equivalent dose = CPZ*	*Half-life*	*Common Side Effect*				
					Sedation	*Weight Gain*	*Sexual dysfunction*	*Anticholi-nergic*	*EPS*
Phenothiazines									
A. Aliphatics									
1. Chlorpromazine	300-1500	50-100	100	16-30	++++	+++	+++	++++	+
2. Triflupromazine	100-400	30-60	25	–	+++	+++	–	+++	++
3. Promazine	40-800	50-150	40	–	++			+++	
B. Piperidines									
1. Thioridazine	300-800	–	100	9-30	++++	+++	+++	++++	+
2. Mesoridazine	100-400	–	50	16-27	++	++	+++	+++	+
C. Piperazines									
1. Trifluperazine	15-60	1-5	5	13h	++	+	++	++	+++
2. Prochloperazine	45-150	40-80	15						+++
3. Fluphenazine	.2-20	—	2	13-58	++	+	++	++	+++
4. Fluphenazine deconate	–	20-50◆◆	***	>16 day	++	+	++	++	+++
Thioxanthenes									
A. Aliphatics									
1. Chlorprothixene	75-600	25-75	50	8-12	+++	+++	+	+	++
B. Piperazines				34h					
1. Thiothixene	6-60	2-6	5	12-28	++	++	+	+	++
2. Zuclopenthixol	25-150	50-100	–			+	++	+++	–
3. Zuclopenthixol decanoate	–	200-400	****	19 day	+++	+	++	++	–
4. Flupenthixol	3-40	–	–	26-36	+	+++	++	++	+++
5. Flupenthixol decanoate	–	20-40◆◆	*****	8-17 day	+	+++	++	++	+
Butyrophenones									
1. Haloperidol	5-100	5-20	2	12-36	+	+++	++	++	+++
2. Haloperidol decanoate	–	25-250	******	12 day	+++	+	+	++	+++
3. Trifluperidol	0.5-0.8		0.6	29-55	++	+	+	+	+++
DiphenylButylPiperidines									
1. Pimozide	4-20	2.5-5.0◆◆	2	+	++	+	++	++	
2. Penfluridol	20-60◆		3.5	6.5	+		+	+	++
Indolic derivatives									
1. Molindone	50-225	–	10	8-30	++	–	NA	+++	+
Dibenzoxazepines									
1. Loxapine	25-100	–	10			–	NA	+++	++
Atypical antipsychotics									
A. Dibenzodiazepines	50-450	–	50	5-16	++++	++++	+	+++	0
1. Clozapine									
B. Substituted Benzamides									
1. Sulpiride	400-1800	–	–	–	++	+++	NA		0
2. Amisulpiride	400-1200	–	–	–	–		NA		±
C. Benzisoxales									
1. Resperidone	2-10	–	1-2	20-24	++	++	+++	++	±
D. Benzisothiazolyl	40-160	–	20	–	+	++	+	++	0
1. Ziprasidone									
Thienobenzodiazepine									
1. Olanzepine	50-20	–	2-3	21-54	++++	++++	++	+++	0
E. Diabenzothiazepine									
1. Quetiapine	300-500	–	50-100	6-7	+++	+	+	+	±

Note: ◆ = Once Every week; ◆◆= Every 2 weeks.

*** = 25 mg of Fluphenazine deconate every 2 weeks =300CPZ/day.

**** = 200 mg of Zuclopenthixol deconate every 2 weeks = 25 mg/day of oral clopixol.

***** = 40 mg of Flupenthixol deconate every 2 weeks = 25 mg of Fluphenazine deconate every 2 weeks.

****** = 100 mg of Haloperidol deconate every 4 weeks = 5 mg/day of oral Haloperidol.

+ = Mild; ++ = Moderate; +++ = Severe; ± = Probably/ Very little; 0 = Absent.

Patient and his family members should be explained about effects, side effects, doses and duration of medications. A patient teaching programme should include the following:

1. The medication regimen and the importance of taking medication as directed.
2. Signs and symptoms of tardive dyskinesia, and instructions to report any incidence to the physician.
3. Effects of noncompliance and the return of symptoms when medications are discontinued.
4. Importance of taking medication with food or milk to decrease stomach irritation.
5. Use of caution when operating motor vehicle and machines.
6. Knowledge of effect, side-effect and doses of psychotropics–not to stop medicine abruptly.
7. Importance of taking medicine.
8. Knowledge of duration needed before full effect of treatment.

ANTIPARKINSONIAN DRUGS

Although these drugs have no direct therapeutic use, yet can be used to control the extra pyramidal side effects of antipsychotic drugs. Commonly used drugs are benztropine mesylate, trihexyphenidyl hydrochloride, procyclidine and orphenadrine. In addition to increasing the likelihood of tardive dyskinesia, anticholinergic side effects can add to those of antipsychotic drug to increase constipation and precipitate glaucoma or urinary retention.

Contraindications

The main contraindications are hypersensitivity reaction of the drug, narrow-angle glaucoma, myasthenia gravis, urinary retention, peptic ulcer disease, prostatic hypertrophy, and children under 3 years of age. These drugs must be used with caution in older people because of significant side effects, including urinary retention, visual disturbance, palpitations, and increased intraocular pressure.

ANTIDEPRESSANT DRUGS

The modern era of the treatment of depression with medication began in the 1950s when ipsoniazid, a Mono Amino oxidase Inhibitors (MAOIs) used for the treatment of tuberculosis, was noted to elevate mood. Imipramine, the first of the tricyclic antidepressant (TCAs), was developed as a derivative of chlorpromazine; it was hoped that imipramine would be more effective than chlorpromazine as an antipsychotic agent. Although imipramine did not show antipsychotic efficacy, it was shown to be effective in the treatment of depression. Subsequently, many more antidepressants have been approved for use. To date, all antidepressant appear to be equally effective for treating major depression. In addition, these medications are significantly different from one another with regard to side effects, lethality in overdose, pharmacokinetics, and the ability to treat co-morbid psychiatric disorders.

With the advancement of pharmacotherapy, TCAs are rarely used these days. Main problem with their use is sleep and weight gain. Drug of choice these days are SSRIs. Other drugs that are quite frequently used because of their benign side effect profile are mirtazapine and bupropion. One important property of these drugs is that they do not cause sexual dysfunctions and may be used for treatment of SSRI induced dysfunctions.

Mechanism of Action

All current antidepressant drugs affect the serotonergic and/or catecholaminergic systems in the central nervous systems (CNS). The effects of antidepressants on monoamine availability are immediate, but the clinical response is typically delayed for several weeks.

Tricyclic Antidepressant Drugs (TCAs)

Most tricyclic antidepressant drugs act through inhibition of the reuptake of norepinephrine, serotonin, and to a lesser extent dopamine. These mechanisms are thought to be responsible for the therapeutic action of tricyclic antidepressants. In addition, TCA block muscarinic cholinergic receptors, H_1 histamine receptors, and α_1 adrenergic receptors. These mechanisms are thought to account for the side effects of the TCAs.

Commonly used TCAs are Imipramine, Amitriptyline, Clomipramine, Tri-imipramine and Doxepine (tertiary amines) and Desipramine, Nortriptyline and Protriptyline (secondary amines).

Risks, Side Effects and Their Management

Anticholinergic side effects: The most common anticholinergic side effects are dry mouth, constipation, urinary retention, blurred vision, and tachycardia. In elderly persons anticholinergic medications may cause cognitive impairment and confusion.

Cholinergic medications have been reported to relieve some of the anticholinergic side effects. Bethanecol chloride may alleviate dry mouth, constipation, urinary hesitancy and retention, erectile and ejaculatory dysfunctions.

Sedation: The relative sedating properties of the TCAs appear to parallel their respective histamine receptor binding affinities. Tri-imipramine, Amitriptyline, and Doxepine are the most sedating TCAs. Desipramine and Protriptyline are less sedating.

Cardiac effects: Many of the TCAs have cardiovascular effects, including orthostatic hypotension and cardiac conduction delays. Orthostatic hypotension is the cardiovascular side effects that most commonly result in serious morbidity, because TCA at toxic level (as occur in overdose) can cause life threatening arrhythmias.

Weight gain: Patients treated with TCAs may experience undesirable weight gain.

Neurological effects: A dose related risk of seizures has been found with Clomipramine. Daily dosage of this drug should not exceed 250 mg.

Allergic reaction: Allergic and hypersensitivity reactions may occur with TCAs, as they may with most drugs.

SEROTONIN SPECIFIC REUPTAKE INHIBITORS (SSRIs)

Since 1988 number of Serotonin Specific Reuptake Inhibitors (SSRIs) like Fluoxetine, Sertraline, and Paroxetine, Escitalopram and Duloxetine have been introduced for the treatment of depression and an additional SSRI, Fluvoxamine, has been approved for the treatment of obsessive compulsive disorder. SSRIs are widely used with other disorders including impulse control disorders, post traumatic stress disorders, borderline personality disorder and eating disorder.

The SSRIs share a common mechanism of action: they potently inhibit the reuptake of serotonin without significant effects on the reuptake of norepinephrine and dopamine. Consequently, SSRIs cause fewer troublesome side effects, such as anticholinergic effects, weight gain, and sedation, than the tricyclic and tetracyclic drugs and are also safer when taken in overdose compared to the tricyclic drugs.

The adverse effects of the SSRIs are similar, although minor pharmacological differences and individual patients sensitivities may result in some patients better tolerating one SSRI than another. Commonly noted side effects include anxiety, insomnia, gastrointestinal symptoms (such as nausea and diarrhea), headache, decreased appetite and sexual dysfunction (such as delayed orgasm and decreased libido). Other adverse effects include lethargy, fatigue, sweating, tremor and other extra pyramidal symptoms. Hyponatremia, elevated cholesterol and prolonged bleeding time may be found on laboratory testing.

Effect of antidepressant drugs on depression is not immediate. They must be taken continuously for several weeks before therapeutic effects are evident.

NURSING MANAGEMENT OF PATIENT

It is evident that role of nurse is significant when caring for the patient on antidepressant drug therapy. Following nursing interventions for patients on antidepressant drug therapy must be included:

- Provide information on drug action and side effects.
- Advise patient to take medication exactly as directed by the psychiatrists and for several weeks to months to see a therapeutic effect.
- Give medication with food or milk to avoid stomach upset.
- Give medication at bed time due to a sedative nature of agents.
- Advise your patient to use caution when driving, operating dangerous equipment or engaging in activities that require alertness and coordination.
- In case of complaint of retention of urine, intake and output of patients should be recorded.
- Monitor vital signs and observe for orthostatic hypotension and advise to change position slowly.
- Monitor mood at frequent intervals.
- Keep a watch for hoarding of drugs and assess for suicidal ideation.
- Record your observation regularly (Side effects) and inform consultant as and when required.

ANTI ANXIETY DRUGS (BENZODIAZEPINES)

These drugs are mainly used for treatment of anxiety disorders or associated anxiety in any illness. Based on the duration of action, benzodiazepines are divided into short acting drugs (Alprazolam, Lorazepam, Oxazepam etc.) and long acting drugs (Chlordiazepoxide, Diazepam, Flurazepam, Clonazepam etc.). Out of these we should use long acting drugs as they have fewer propensities for dependence due to absence of withdrawal symptoms. However they are contraindicated in elderly patients because of slow clearance. In addition to anxiolytic, sedative, hypnotic they also have muscle relaxant and anticonvulsant properties. Benzodiazepines should be used only when it is indicated. The use should be for a short period such as 3-4 weeks.

Side Effects

Main side effects of benzodiazepines are drowsiness, ataxia, disturbed concentration, and impairment of driving skills. Benzodiazepines should be avoided in the first trimester of pregnancy.

Withdrawal Effects

Withdrawal symptoms may occur in more than 50% patients after a prolonged use of more than six months. The symptoms are usually noticed after 2-3 days of discontinuation of drug and persist for a few weeks. They include insomnia, tremors, irritability, increased sensitivity to stimuli, muscle twitching and occasionally seizures.

NURSING MANAGEMENT

Role of nurse taking care of patients who is on anti-anxiety medication include the following interventions:

- Be aware of side effects and potential adverse effects.

- Give medication with food or milk to prevent nausea and vomiting.
- Monitor lying and standing blood pressure daily.
- Instruct the patient to avoid driving or operating dangerous machinery while taking the drug.
- Advise the patient not to discontinue taking drug abruptly. Abrupt withdrawal can be life-threatening. (Symptoms may include depression, anxiety, abdominal and muscle cramps, tremors, insomnia, vomiting, diaphoresis, convulsions, and delirium).
- Instruct the patient not to drink alcohol or take other CNS depressants while taking these drugs.
- Assess patient's mood and orientation daily.
- In case patients complain of sleep disturbance the causable factor should be identified and a calm and quiet environment should be provided.

MOOD STABILIZERS

Mood stabilizing drugs are used in the treatment of mania and as prophylaxis in recurrent mood disorder. The most commonly used drugs in this category are (i) Lithium, (ii) Carbamazepine, and (iii) Sodium valproate. The choice is mostly empirical however certain principles may help in deciding the drug. Frequent and severe depressive episodes call for the use of Carbamazepine. Patients with euphoric mania, positive family history, manic depressive illness pattern responds better to Lithium whereas multiple episodes, rapid cycling, and dysphoric mania, and depressive manic illness pattern responds well to Valproate. Other putative mood stabilizer is Lamotrigine.

LITHIUM

It is the lightest of alkali metals and is a monovalent ion. It is available as carbonate for oral use. The therapeutic and toxic doses are close to each other, so it is essential to measure plasma concentrations of lithium at regular intervals. The measurement should be made first weekly for 3-4 weeks; and then biweekly and then once in a month provided that a satisfactory steady state has been achieved. The timing of the measurement is important and is normally measured 12 hours after the last dose. The usually recommended plasma concentration for the treatment of acute mania is 0.8 to 1.2 mmol/litre and for prophylaxis of recurrent mood disorder is 0.4 to 0.8 mmol/litre.

Side Effects

Early side effects include diuresis, tremor, dry mouth, metallic taste, weakness and fatigue. Later effects include fine tremor, polyuria and polydipsia, thyroid enlargement, hypothyroidism, impaired memory and ECG changes.

Long Term Effects

1. *Effects on kidney:* This can lead to dehydration with the risk of lithium intoxication with polyuria or dehydration. Patient should be advised to drink enough water to compensate for the fluid loss. A few patients develop nephrogenic diabetes insipidus due to interference with the effect of antidiuretic hormone. Renal functions should therefore be checked every six months.
2. *Tremors:* Tremors occur frequently, and if this is troublesome, propanolol may be used to reduce the symptom. Coarse tremor is a sign of toxicity.
3. *Thyroid:* About 5% of patients taking lithium develop hypothyroidism with a compensatory rise in thyroid stimulating hormone.
4. *Toxic effects of lithium:* Toxic effects of lithium are nausea, vomiting, diarrhoea, coarse tremor, ataxia, dysarthria, muscle twitching,

Table 25.2: Antidepressant drugs

Class and Oral Name of Drug	*Dose*	*Half Life (hr)*	*Common Side Effect*			
			Sedation	*Sexual Dysfunction*	*Wt. Gain*	*Anticholinergic*
TCAs (Group)						
(5-HT+NE reuptake inhibition)						
A. **Tertiary amine**	75-300	7.6	++	++++	+++	+++
1. Imipramine	75-300	26.6	++++	++	++++	++++
2. Amtriptyline	75-300	16.8	++++	++	+++	++
3. Doxepine	75-300	24	++	+	++	++
4. Tri-Imipramine	75-300	32	++	++++	+++	+++
5. Clomipramine	75-250	–	+++	++	+++	+++
6. Dotheipin	75-300					
B. **Secondary Amine**						
1. Nortriptyline	75-200	26.6	++	–	+	+
2. Protriptyline	15-60	78.4	0	–	+–	++
3. Desipramine	75-300	17.1	+	–	+	++
C. **Bicyclic antidepressant**						
1. Viloxazine	100-300		+	NA	NA	+
D. **Tetracyclic antidepressants**						
1. Mianserin	30-120		+++	+	++	+
2. Maprotiline	75-225	43.3	++	+	+++	++
3. Amoxepine	150-400		++	+	+++	++
SSRIs (Group)						
(5-HTreuptake inhibit.)						
1. Fluoxetine	10-60	72	Activating	++++	–	0
2. Paroxetine	10-40	20	++	++++	+	0
3. Fluvoxamine	15-300	15	+	++++	+	+
4. Sertraline	20-200	26	+	++++	+	0
5. Citalopram	10-40	35	+	++	++	0
SNRIs (Group)						
(5-HT+NE>DA reuptake inhib.)						
1. Vanlafexine	75-375	15	+	+++	+	+
NaSSA (Group)						
(α_2 **Adrenergic+5HT$_2$ antag.**)						
1. Mirtazepine	15-45	20-40	++++	+	++++	+
NDRIs (Group)						
(DA+NE reuptake inhibition)						
1. Bupropion	15-450	12-14	Activating	–	+–	0
SARIs (Group)						
(DA+NE reuptake inhibition)						
1. Trazodone	150-600	4-9	++++	–	NA	+
2. Nefazodone	200-600	5-15	++	–	NA	+
NARIs (Group)						
(selective NE reuptake inhibiti.)						
1. Reboxetine	8-10	–	±	+	NA	+
MAOIs (Group)						
(Inhibit monoamine oxidase)						
1. Selegiline	5-10	2-3		NA	NA	
2. Moclobemide	300-600	1-3	Activating	NA	NA	0

Abbreviation: + = Mild; ++ = Moderate; +++ = Severe; ± = Rarely; 0 = Absent; NA = Not available hyper reflexia, confusion, coma, convulsion, renal failure and cardiovascular collapse (See Table).

Management

Lithium toxicity is a medical emergency because it can progress through coma and lead to death. Most patients recover completely, few survive with permanent neurological damage (See Table).

Teratogenesis

Lithium crosses the placenta and, there are reports of increased rates of fatal abnormalities particularly affecting the heart. Drug should be avoided in first trimester of pregnancy.

Contraindications

Contraindications include renal failure or recent renal disease, cardiac failure or recent myocardial infarction, chronic diarrhea sufficient to alter electrolyte levels.

CARBAMAZEPINE

Carbamazepine, primarily used as an anticonvulsant, has been found to be effective in the prophylaxis of recurrent mood disorder. It is effective in some patients unresponsive to lithium, and for some with rapidly recurring manic depressive disorder. Dosage is similar to that for epilepsy 800-3000 mg/day. Side effects include drowsiness, dizziness, nausea, double vision and skin rash. A rare but serious side effect is agranulocytosis.

SODIUM VALPROATE

Like carbamazepine, sodium valproate is an anticonvulsant that has been found to prevent the recurrence of bipolar disorder, especially in patients who do not respond to lithium or carbamazepine.

Common side effects include sedation, tiredness, tremor and gastrointestinal disturbance. Sodium valproate may cause other unwanted effects including thrombocytopenia.

Table 25.3: Signs and symptoms of lithium toxicity

Mild to Moderate intoxication (Lithium Level = 1.5-2.0 mEq/L)	
Gastrointestinal	Vomiting Abdominal Pain Dryness of Mouth
Neurological	Ataxia Dizziness Slurred speech Nystagmus Lethargy or Excitement Muscle Weakness
Moderate to Severe Intoxication (Lithium Level = 2.0-2.5 mEq/L)	
Gastrointestinal	Anorexia Persistent nausea and vomiting
Neurological	Blurred Vision Muscle fasciculation Clonic limb movements Hyperactive deep tendon reflexes Choreoathetoid movements Convulsions Delirium Syncope Electroencephalographic changes Stupor Coma Circulatory Failure (lowered blood pressure, Cardiac arrhythmias and conduction abnormalities)
Severe Lithium Intoxication (Lithium level>2.5 mEq/L)	
	Generalized convulsion Oliguria and renal failure. Death

Contraindications

The main contraindications are hypersensitivity to the drug, cardiac or renal disease, sodium imbalance, and pregnancy and lactation. It should be used cautiously in older people and those with metabolic disorders, urinary retention, or seizure disorders. The action of anticonvulsants and calcium channel blockers in the treatment of bipolar disorder is not clear. However, they have been used effectively to stabilize the manic episodes in bipolar disorders.

NURSING MANAGEMENT OF PATIENT

Nursing interventions during planning care for the patients receiving mood stabilizers include:

Nursing Diagnosis

Nursing diagnosis applicable to the patient receiving a mood-stabilizing agent may include:

- Risk for injury, related to side effects of drowsiness and dizziness.
- Risk for violence, related to manic excitement, impulsive behavior.
- Risk for poisoning, related to lithium toxicity (narrow therapeutic range of drug).
- Risk for dehydration, related to side effects of medication (nausea, vomiting, and diarrhea).
- Sensory/perceptual disturbances, related to chemical alterations.
- Self-esteem, related to perceived lack of control.

Nursing Interventions

Following nursing actions should be included, while planning care for the patient receiving mood-stabilizing drugs.

- Teach patient and his/her family about mood-stabilizing drug therapy.
- Educate the patient to look for expected side effects of the drug without creating anxiety. Teach the patient about possible side effects likely to appear such as nausea, dry mouth, flatulence, dizziness, mild tremors, and insomnia and tell him that they subside with continued treatment.
- Administer medication with food to avoid nausea and dyspepsia.
- Fluid intake must be about 2000 to 3000 ml daily.
- Assess for signs of toxicity in the patient taking lithium carbonate therapy.
- Inform the physician of any indication of lithium toxicity.
- Report any symptom of drug side effects to the physician.
- Do not stop taking the drug abruptly-serious withdrawal symptoms can occur.
- Take medication regularly, even when feeling well.
- Take medication at the same time each day. If a dose is missed, do not double the dose the next time (could result in toxicity).
- Report any mood swings or extreme changes in mood to the physician.
- For patient taking lithium instruct him to increase fluid intake.

KEY POINTS

- Chlorpromazine was first neuroleptic introduced in 1950.
- Antipsychotics are divided into Typical (conventional) and Atypical antipsychotic drugs.
- Conventional antipsychotic drugs act by blocking dopaminergic receptors mainly present in meso-limbic system (antipsychotic effect) and extra pyramidal system (Extra pyramidal side effects).
- Atypical antipsychotic drugs particularly act on the 5-HT2 receptors.

- Extra pyramidal side effects include Akathisia, Acute dystonia, Parkinsonian syndrome, Tardive dyskinesia, Neuroleptic malignant syndrome and Rabbit syndrome (peri-oral tremors).
- Most common extra pyramidal side effect is Akathisia.
- Anticholinergic side effects include dry mouth, constipation, urinary retention, orthostatic hypotension, mydrisis and sexual problems.
- All antipsychotics are equally efficacious, but differ in side effect profile.
- Atypical antipsychotics are effective antipsychotics without or with least extra pyramidal side effects.
- Atypical antipsychotics available in Indian market are Clozapine, Risperidone, Olanzapine, Ziprasidone and Quetiapine.
- Agranulocytosis is serious side effect of Clozapine.
- Most Atypical antipsychotics causes weight gain.
- Depot Preparations are given to those who are not compliant with daily oral medication. Available preparations are Fluphenazine decanoate, Flupenthixol decanoate, haloperidol decanoate, Zuclopenthixol decanoate.
- The usually recommended plasma concentration of lithium for the treatment of acute mania is 0.8 to 1.2 mmol/litre and for prophylaxis of recurrent mood disorder is 0.4 to 0.8 mmol/litre.
- Imipramine was first antidepressant discovered by Kuhn in 1958.
- Antidepressants are classified in 4 major classes (a) Cyclic antidepressants (b) SSRIs (c) MAOI (d) Other newer antidepressants.
- SSRIs include Fluoxetine, Fluvoxamine, Paroxetine, Sertoraline, Citalopram, and Escitalopram.
- SSRIs are devoid of troublesome sedation and anticholinergic side effects, hence consider as first line of drugs for management of depression.
- Reversible MAO-B inhibitors are selegiline (antiparkinsonian also) and moclobemide. They do not carry the risk of hypertensive crisis.
- Therapeutic level of lithium above 1.5 meq/L produces toxicity.
- GI side effects are the most common short term side effects with lithium whereas most common long term side effects are renal.
- The most common lithium induced EEG changes is T wave flattening.
- Lithium is absolutely contraindicated in pregnancy first trimester (Ebstein's anomaly common) lactation, psoriasis, CRF, Myasthenia, Hypothyroidism and Addison's disease.
- Nurse must be well versed with the effects, side effects, contraindications, doses and accurate route of psychotropic medications.
- Most antipsychotic cause drowsiness. Medicine should be administered at bed time. The patient should be advised not to drive and handle heavy machinery while taking antipsychotic.
- Nurse should be well versed with extrapyramidal side effects of antipsychotic drugs. Nurse should monitor the patient for extrapyramidal side effects. An early observation, reporting and use of anti parkinsonian drugs can reduce the side effects of these medicines.
- Patient and his family members should be explained about effects, side effects, doses and duration of medications. A patient teaching programme must include all these informations.

- Advise patient to take medication exactly as directed by the psychiatrists and for several weeks to months to see a therapeutic effect.
- Record your observation regularly (Side effects) and inform consultant as and when required.
- Keep a watch for hoarding of drugs and assess for suicidal ideation.

B. ECT AND OTHER BIOLOGICAL THERAPIES

ELECTROCONVULSIVE THERAPY (ECT)

Prompted by the observation that occurrence of spontaneous seizure in patients with schizophrenia led to improvement in their psychotic state, Von Meduna in 1934 used injections of camphor to induce seizures and showed benefits of such a treatment in psychotic symptoms. Later, because of erratic and unpredictable nature of response of camphor other substances were tried.

Cerletti and Bini in 1938 in Rome were the first to use electrical shock to induce seizures for the treatment of psychosis. At first this treatment was called electroshock therapy (EST) but later on its name was changed to electroconvulsive therapy (ECT).

Electroconvulsive therapy (ECT) is one of the most effective treatment methods in psychiatry. Because of misinformation about ECT and the stigma attached with its application in the patients, ECT is underused. Due to improvements in the techniques of administration of anesthesia as well as improvements in delivery of electrical current to the patient, ECT is now regarded as a safe procedure that is effective yet devoid of irreversible or hazardous side effects.

Mechanism of Action

The exact mechanism of action of ECT is not known. It is now well accepted that induction of bilateral generalized seizure is essential for the beneficial effects of ECT. Research indicates that application of ECT leads to change in almost all neurotransmitter system and this is in some way responsible for the beneficial effects of ECT.

Indications

Following are the major indications of ECT:

1. **Major depressive disorder with risk of suicide:** This is the most frequently cited indication for the use of ECT. In this disorder, ECT is considered to be the fastest and most effective mode of treatment available.
2. **Acute manic episodes:** If patient is excited or for some reason pharmacotherapy cannot be instituted or has to be discontinued.
3. Schizophrenia with marked catatonic feature.

Clinical Application of ECT

The mention of ECT in management often generates considerable anxiety and apprehension in patients and their caregivers; therefore, it is important that the matter of administration of ECT as a method of treatment must be discussed in detail with the patients and their caregivers to relieve their fears, concerns and misconception about ECT. A written informed consent must be obtained and in the process of obtaining informed consent, adequate information about the need for ECT, the nature of the treatment, the possible numbers of ECT, the procedure involved and possible side effects must be given in understandable language to the patient and the caregivers.

Procedure

The ECT procedure consists of the following:

1. **Pre ECT evaluation:** Before giving ECT to the patient, a thorough physical and neurological examination, laboratory investigations (like haemogram, blood biochemistry, urine analysis, X-ray chest, ECG), pre anesthetic

check-up for suitability to receive anesthesia and dental examination to check loose tooth is to be performed. Pre-treatment evaluation is necessary to establish that the patient is physically fit to receive anesthesia and ECT. Dental check-up is essential so that loose tooth if any can be detected, the presence of which can create a hazardous situation during ECT induced seizure as a loose tooth can get dislodged in respiratory passage and choke the patient.

2. **Pre anesthetic medications:** The patient should be fasting overnight. Anticholinergic medication (Atropine 0.6-1 mg i.v.) should be given in the morning to reduce secretions. Anesthesia is generally induced by giving a short-acting agent such as thiopental or methoexital (2.5-5% solution) by IV route. Succinylcholine (0.5 mg/ kg), a short acting muscle relaxant agent, is generally preferred to induce muscle relaxation.
3. **Electrode placement for ECT:** Use of Bilateral placement of electrodes is the usual practice. Bifrontotemporal positioning of the electrodes is the most common site of electrodes placement. In a few cases, unilateral placement (non-dominant hemisphere) is recommended to avoid post- ECT confusion or if the patient is elderly. Brief pulse waveform of electrical stimulation is the most prevalent form of current with modern ECT machines.
4. **ECT induced seizure:** Initially when ECT was used as a direct method (e.g. electric shock was given to a conscious patient (direct ECT)), the induced seizure were similar to a generalized tonic clonic seizures. Later on when anesthesia was combined with muscle relaxant (modified ECT) to make the procedure safe and free of side effects particularly bone fractures, the administration of muscle relaxant makes it difficult to monitor manifestation of seizure activity. However, to be sure that seizure has been induced, either a cuff method can be used or advantage can be taken of modern machines which have inbuilt facility of EEG and/or EMG recording. It is generally accepted that for ECT treatment to be effective, the duration of induced seizure should be at least for 25 seconds. To measure the duration of seizure by cuff method isolate one arm by inflating the cuff to above systolic blood pressure before the muscle relaxant is given. It will not be paralyzed by succinylcholine and show twitching.
5. **Post ECT recovery:** Patient should be oxygenated, because of administration of muscle relaxant. Once spontaneous breathing is established, the patient should be nursed ensuing patency of airway and freedom from inhalation of secretions. Vital signs monitoring should be done. Usually the patients recover in 20-30 minutes.

Side Effects

The common adverse effects of ECT are headache, confusion and short lasting delirium following recovery from the seizures:

The patients also have short lasting memory impairment that is completely reversible over a period of time. The other side effects such as bone fractures are common in direct ECT method, but now rarely occur due to the use of muscle relaxants during the course of ECT. The mortality rate with ECT is very low and it is a safe and non-hazardous treatment modality.

Contraindications

There is no absolute contraindication to use of ECT, except raised intracranial pressure. ECT should be used with extreme caution in advanced pregnancy, in patients with intracranial space occupying lesions, patients with recent myocardial infraction, severe hypertension and retinal detachment.

ROLE OF NURSE IN ECT TREATMENT

The psychiatric patients are most frequently hospitalized for ECT treatment, though some of the out patients are also given ECT treatment.

Hospital Setting

In a hospital setting where the electroconvulsive therapy is given, the nurse should see to the set-up which includes:

1. Waiting room or resting room.
2. Treatment room or ECT room.
3. Recovery room or after-care room.

1. **Waiting room or resting room:** In this room patients are asked to wait or take rest before electroconvulsive therapy. The room should be calm with dim lights, light color of the walls. Put some flowers to give pleasant feelings to the patient. There should be some magazines to read, so that the patient can divert his mind and reduce anxiety. Lavatory (toilet) should be attached, because the patient needs to empty his bladder and bowels before getting ECT. The nurse should always be available in this room so that the patient and relatives can clarify their doubts. Preanasthetic drug should be kept ready.
2. **Treatment room/ECT room:** In the treatment room the nurse needs to do the following preparations:

   Articles for comfort of the patient: The room should be near the waiting room. For privacy a bedside screen, well-padded low level beds with railings should be placed to prevent injury due to fall.

   Articles for preparation of the patient: Small pillows should be put under the patients waist to prevent injury. Use mouth gag to prevent injury to the tongue during convulsions and to keep the airway patent. Tongue spatula, endotracheal tube and sterile catheter (for suction of the respiratory tract), O_2 cylinder and an ambu bag (to give oxygen immediately after the therapy and to give artificial respiration, if required) must be ready for use.

   Articles for the procedure: A trolly with an ECT machine in working order, Jelly or normal saline for putting on electrodes (as normal saline is a good conductor of electricity and it facilitates in passing current), Emergency drugs and a resuscitation tray, B.P. apparatus, sterile syringes and spirit swabs must be kept ready for use. Check all the electric plug points and ensure adequate light in room. Doctor and nurse should be present in the ECT room.
3. **Recovery room or after-care room:** Once the patient responds to a painful stimulus he is transferred to the recovery room. A floor bed with 1 to 1½" padding on the sides for the patients should be kept ready. Observation of vital signs and symptoms such as B.P., temperature, pulse and respiration should be maintained. An extra sets of clothes in case the patient has spoiled them with urine or faeces during convulsions should be kept ready. Toilet facilities should be available in the recovery room. Once the patient becomes oriented he can be transferred to his ward.

Nursing Interventions

Electroconvulsive therapy involves a significant responsibility for the nursing personnel. Nursing care can be explained as:

A. The patients care before giving ECT.
B. The patient's care during ECT, and
C. The patient's care after ECT.

A. **Nursing Interventions before giving ECT:**

1. Check that a thorough physical examination (heart including ECG, lungs, bone, blood for Hb, urine for sugar and other tests and albumin, and X-rays) is completed.

2. Take written consent or declaration for the treatment from the nearest relative after explaining the method of treatment and risks. Relatives should be told everything in detail.
3. The patient should be empty stomach before treatment. If he is to be treated in an emergency situation, it should be two or three hours after breakfast or meals as it prevents vomiting and aspiration during treatment.
4. Remove artificial dentures.
5. Remove jewellery articles, watch and other thing from his or her body.
6. Remove lipstick, nail polish or any other make-up for easy check of cynosis.
7. Loosen the tight clothes like necktie in men and blouse or other tight garments in women, preferably give hospital clothes.
8. Encourage the patient to empty his bladder and bowels before the treatment to prevent spoiling of bed during treatment.
9. Encourage the patient to maintain his personal hygiene. Remove oil from hair.
10. Give premedication to the patient, Injection Atropine and Diazepam as prescribed by consultant.
11. Take him or her to waiting room.

B. **Nursing Interventions during ECT:**

1. After transfer to the ECT room on a well-padded bed, place in a comfortable dorsal position or supine position. A small pillow is placed under the lumber curve.
2. Give a short acting anesthetic agent. Thiopental 0.25gm to 0.5gms. I/V, and Scoline (Succinylcholine) 30 to 50 mgm. (Check prescription). The doses of drugs may vary from patient to patient.
3. Well-padded mouth gag or tongue depressor is placed in between the teeth.
4. Keep head in hyperextension state with support to chin to prevent jaw dislocation and to keep airway patent.
5. Give a few breaths of oxygen to the patient to support phase of apnea after convulsions.
6. Provide electrodes dipped in saline water or jelly for placing on the temporal region, because saline is a good conductor of electricity.
7. Make an observation of grand mal seizures. The presence of the initial tonic stage which lasts for 10-15 seconds, followed by convulsions lasting for 25 to 30 seconds.
8. Do suction immediately to prevent aspiration.
9. Restore respiration by giving oxygen by mask, if required.

Nursing Interventions after ECT

- Record the pulse, respiration and blood pressure of the patient, regularly till they are stabilized.
- Transfer the patient to the recovery room only when he or she can respond to your commands.
- Allow the patient to sleep for 30 minutes to one hour, if he/she wants to sleep.
- Reassurance to the patient and reorient the patient to the ward, toilet and nurse's station.
- Make a note of any injuries or complaints of pain by the patient-body pain or headache.
- Encourage the patient to take a bath and change his/her clothes and help the patient to carry on his daily activities as planned. He should be allowed to go to the day-care room.

KEY POINTS

- Von Meduna in 1934 used injections of camphor to induce seizures and showed benefits of such a treatment in psychotic symptoms.
- Cerletti and Bini in 1938 in Rome were the first to use electrical shock to induce seizures for the treatment of psychosis.
- Indications for ECT are Major depression with suicidal ideation, acutely excited manic patients and catatonic patients.
- ECT is given as 80-120 volts for 0.2-0.8 seconds.
- Headache, confusion and reversible memory loss are common side effects of ECT.
- There is no absolute contraindication to use of ECT, except raised intracranial pressure.
- Electroconvulsive therapy involves a significant responsibility of the nursing personnel. Nursing care can be explained as:
  1. The patient's care before giving ECT.
  2. The patient's care during ECT, and
  3. The patient's care after ECT.

C. PSYCHOLOGICAL METHODS OF TREATMENT

In addition to pharmacology there are other non-pharmacological methods that are important to practice in the treatment of patients in psychiatry. These include psychotherapy and behavior therapies.

Psychotherapy is described as a dialogue between a mental health professional and the patient with a goal of reducing the symptoms of the emotional disturbance or disorder and improving the individual's personal and social well being. The aim of this dialogue is not to give advice, but to allow patients to learn about themselves, their life and their feelings and to make choices toward changes. The intent is for patients to rediscover their own person, their priorities and inner courage to act on them.

Depending upon the goals and primary methods these can be divided into following types:

1. Psychoanalytic psychotherapy.
2. Group psychotherapy.
3. Time limited psychotherapies.
4. Cognitive behavior therapy.

The choice of a particular therapy depends upon nature and severity of patient's illness, his expectation with the treatment, willingness for therapy, frustration tolerance, time available for treatment, and therapist's skill.

1. PSYCHOANALYTIC PSYCHOTHERAPY

This psychotherapeutic approach is primarily based on Sigmund Freud's work. It is aimed at partial personality reorganization by uncovering the conflicts and maladaptive defense mechanisms. For it, patient must be psychological minded, i.e., he must be able to understand the cause for his behavior and must have insight and wish to change his maladaptive behaviors.

Once therapist and patient, both find each other's acceptance, therapeutic relationship (alliance) is established. This therapy lasts for up to 3-5 years and 1-3 sessions/week are held. The patient is asked to sit face to face with therapist and his current life issues are dealt. Depending upon the patient's needs, therapist may use supportive techniques and interpretation and clarification of the products of analysis. Liberal use of medication is acceptable during therapy.

2. GROUP PSYCHOTHERAPY

In this method the therapeutic approach is directed towards a group. This is a group of people with similar problems, similar needs and they share the similar interventional requirements. Joseph Pratt is credited as the founder of this method.

The success of group interaction depends upon the degree of trust, openness and interpersonal risk taking among the members. Groups of people with substance abuse (Alcohol anonymous), AIDS etc have gained popularity. Groups can also be formed on short term basis e.g., during natural calamities, disaster, bereavement, medical problems etc.

First step is the formation of a group that is usually done by the therapist, the size of dynamically oriented group is 6-10 people. The duration of meetings is 75-120 minutes, mostly once a week. There should be ample space and the members have a liberty to choose their seat. The members must be strong in ego, should have motivation to change, must posses insight and must have history of satisfying relationships. Then members work together to explore intrapsychic conflicts and their resolution under the guidance of skilled therapist.

The therapist is the leader of the group and is supposed to understand the emotional needs of members of the group and guide them in a smooth manner so that they start working with each other.

3. TIME LIMITED PSYCHOTHERAPIES

In this method time frame is pre-decided that can last for 1-40 sessions (Commonly 12-20 sessions) and there after therapy is terminated. They are not useful for long lasting character problems but can be used for oedipal conflicts, mood, anxiety and eating disorders.

Following techniques can be used for therapy in this domain:

i. **Interpersonal therapy:** Focus of the therapy is poor interpersonal relationships. The dynamics or cause for conflict is not addressed; rather the focus of treatment is interpersonal relationships.
   The patient is guided to behave in a socially acceptable manner that can change other persons view regarding him, thus leading to better relationships.
ii. **Cognitive behavior therapy:** The aim of the therapy is to identify the distorted thoughts that lead to maladaptive behavior and feelings. The patient is asked to find out negative automatic thoughts and relaxation exercises are taught. Described later on.
iii. **Brief psychodynamic psychotherapy:** All the principles described in the section of psychodynamic psychotherapy apply here. The difference is that of duration of treatment, and the central issue that has current importance and past relevance is selected for intervention.

4. COGNITIVE BEHAVIOR THERAPY

The basic principle of the cognitive behavior therapy is: In an (a) adverse situation patient's (b) self image or cognition gets disturbed that leads to (c) maladaptive feelings (Depression and Anxiety) which in turn lead to (d) maladaptive behavior pattern further leading to (a) adverse situation.

This therapy focuses on identifying and correcting distorted thinking patterns that can lead to emotional distress and problem behaviors. Cognitive therapists believe that patients change their behavior by changing their maladaptive thinking about themselves and their experiences. Patients are taught problem solving skills and stress reducing methods. The important elements of cognitive behavior therapy are as follows:

i. **Cognitive restructuring:** This disturbed cognition originates due to the negative automatic thoughts that come to a person's mind in these situations. These **automatic negative thoughts** can be in the form of- Overgeneralization: This happens with me every time; Maximizing: I have committed a big mistake (after a trivial mistake); Minimizing: I am not going to be affected by this wrong move (after a blunder); and Personalization: Taking a generalized negative event as indicative of negative aspect of self; The therapy starts with the patients' motivation and psychoeducation to the patient regarding these thoughts. He is then asked to maintain a diary of negative automatic thoughts.

   Therapist explains to him the negative thoughts, modifies them into the rational thoughts. Gradually patient learns to overcome dysfunctional thoughts and replaced them with rational thoughts by himself and notes the outcome. A positive outcome, as experienced by patient himself leads him to act on rational thoughts. This is useful in depression, schizophrenia (but not in exacerbations), anxiety disorders, eating disorders etc.

ii. **Time management:** In this method patients are taught to manage their time in such a manner that provides them maximum outcome. The steps are as follows:
   - Set up the priority.
   - Make a schedule of week based on that week's priority.
   - Make a daily schedule based on that day's priority.
   - Allocate the time for every activity.
   - Try to accomplish the goals within allocated time frame.
   - After a review, plan next schedule and work through all stages.

iii. **Problem solving technique:** This method is useful to those patients who are unable to take the decisions in the daily life.

   The essential steps are:
   - Find out the issue and ascertain its importance as a problem to be addressed.
   - Brain storming (Find out all possible alternatives/solutions of problem from personal and other past experiences).
   - Find which is the best alternative to work upon in the present context.
   - Act on that alternative.
   - Note the progress periodically.
   - Review after completion of your act.
   - If the same problem still persists go back to step 3 and if the problem is overcome keep the solution in your mind for future use.

iv. **Social skill training:** In this technique social skills e.g., dressing, meeting people, greeting, talking to them etc. are taught to patients who lack them. The principle is that effective social relationships require reciprocity, respect for another's opinion, appropriate modulation of self disclosure, the ability to yield on some occasions while set limits on others etc. Imperfect social handling leads to stressful experiences. The method employed are modeling (therapist demonstrates more effective alternative approach), role-playing (as in drama) behavior rehearsal etc.

v. **Breathing exercises:** In breathing training patient is trained to take deep slow, rhythmic predominant diaphragmatic breathing during anxiety and hyperventilation episodes that have a calming effect.

vi. **Desensitization:** Systemic desensitization relies on exposure through a progressive hierarchy of fear inducing situations. In this technique fearful situations are coupled with relaxation techniques e.g., exposing a patient of acrophobia to first floor then second and so on. This is useful in phobia, panic attacks and generalized anxiety disorder.

vii. **Flooding:** In this technique instead of progressive hierarchy, maximally anxiety producing stimulus is exposed to patient suddenly resulting in intense anxiety reaction. It supposedly leads to exhaustion of anxiety producing chemicals in brain making the patient fearless e.g., exposing the patient of acrophobia to the top floor.

viii. **Thought stopping:** This is used for the treatment of obsessions. The brain is made to learn through rehearsals the presence of ruminations that are followed by a mental image of STOP or a tap on the table that brings the presence of such behavior to patient's consciousness. The patient then distracts his attention.

ix. **Exposure and response prevention:** In this method, compulsive patient is exposed to anxiety provoking situation and his anxiety generated responses are prevented by relaxing him through above mentioned techniques. For example a patient with OCD of contamination is asked to touch various articles in home that induce anxiety coupled with relaxation. This is based on de-learning and re-learning principle.

x. **Biofeedback methods:** As the name implies, in this method, biological activities of the patient (Pulse, Respiration, Muscle tone, Temperature etc) are shown directly to the patient through the use of machines. A stressful situation is created in the laboratory with the patient and his above parameters are recorded and demonstrated. Then he is made to relax and again same parameters are recorded and change in them is shown to the patient. This helps in patient's understanding of affecting his body physiology through emotions and he can be motivated to stay calm. This can be coupled with all the above procedures.

Role of Nurse

Nurse plays pivotal role in psychological methods of treatment. Nurse's daily interaction with the patient in a healthy therapeutic atmosphere facilitates proper assessment and evaluation of behaviors. The nurse serves as a model for the patient in appropriate social and interactive skills, while reinforcing and rewarding this behavior in the patient. Nurse also helps in conducting various type of therapies like group, family, play or recreational therapy. A psychiatric nurse is an important part of therapeutic process in which recovery and rehabilitation of the patient is facilitated.

KEY POINTS

- Free association, Resistance, Transference and Interpretations are important issues in psychoanalysis.
- Psychotherapy is most indicated in depression, neurotic disorders and personality disorders and not indicated in acute psychosis, organic psychosis and unmotivated patients.
- Cognitive therapy was developed by Aaron Beck and used for treatment of depression, anxiety disorders, phobias, panic disorders and problems of bereavement, divorce etc.
- Group therapy was founded by Joseph Pratt and is helpful in a group of people with similar problems, similar needs and they share the similar interventional requirements (Group of the obese, alcoholics or addicts).

- Classical conditioning is production of conditioned response in relation to conditioned stimulus, given by Ivan P Pavlov.
- B.F.Skinner gave operant conditioning, which is production of a reinforcer to any stimulus or event which when produced by a response, makes that response more likely to occur in future.
- Type of behavior therapy used in different disorders are:

Phobia	:	Desensitization and flooding
Obsession	:	Thought stooping
Compulsion	:	Exposure and response prevention
Anxiety disorder	:	Cognitive restructuring and Muscular exercise
Sexual deviance	:	Aversion therapy
Schizophrenia	:	Token economy

- Biofeedback a is useful mode of therapy for psychosomatic disorders, headache etc.
- In ***Social Skill Training*** patient's social skills like dressing, meeting people, greeting, talking to them etc. are taught to patients who lack them. It is useful in schizophrenia, mental retardation, personality problems.
- Nurse's daily interaction with patient in a healthy therapeutic atmosphere facilitates proper assessment and evaluation of behaviors.
- The nurse serves as a model for the patient in appropriate social and interactive skills.
- Nurse helps in conducting various types of therapies like group, family, play or recreational therapy.

26

Psychiatric Emergencies

DEFINITION

A psychiatric emergency is a psychiatric condition which calls for immediate therapeutic intervention, and is characterized by danger to self or to others (homicidal or destructive acts). It is extremely distressing to the patient and others. Psychiatric emergence may arise in a person with known psychiatric illness, and/or as a complication of some physical illness, injury or drugs. It may arise in a healthy person out of severe stress.

EPIDEMIOLOGY

It is difficult to give prevalence figures, since psychiatric emergencies are seen in diverse situations. The number of emergency patients seen in psychiatric practice is on the increase due to various reasons e.g. deinstitutionalization of psychiatric patients, increase of violence in the society, increased appreciation of the role of organic factors in behaviors, and increasing abuse of alcohol, psychotropic substances and other drugs of abuse.

Psychiatric emergency services are used more by men than women (M:F : 3:2). More visits occur during night hours.

TYPES OF PSYCHIATRIC EMERGENCIES

A large proportion of patients attending emergency room are involuntary. Patients are usually referred from other hospital services, brought by police, relations or voluntary organizations. Common psychiatric emergencies are as follows:

- Violence or excitement
- Suicide
- Delirium
- Panic attacks
- Stupor
- Alcohol or drug intoxication
- Drug withdrawal syndrome
- Social and personal crisis situations.

A number of medical/surgical conditions may also be present as psychiatric emergencies.

Assessment

In all psychiatric emergencies (except the dystonic reaction) aggression to self or others form the common denominator and constitutes the maximum threat. The primary goal of an emergency psychiatric evaluation is the timely assessment of the patient in crisis. The complete assessment includes detailed history taking from informant and patient, evaluation of psychosocial stress, mental status examination, physical assessment of patient with relevent laboratory investigations. Emergency evaluation should address the following questions on priority:

- Is it safe for the patient to be kept in the emergency room?
- Is the patient psychotic?
- Is there any suicidal or homicidal risk?

- What are the immediate needs of the patient?

After the complete work up a provisional diagnosis is made and necessary treatment is started.

VIOLENCE

Violent behavior is a common psychiatric emergency seen in psychiatric clinic. Although majority of mentally ill patients are not dangerous for society or self but some exhibit violent and assaultive behavior with angry outbursts.

Causes of Excited and Violent Behavior

Violence can be due to wide range of psychiatric disorders including:

- Psychotic disorders–Schizophrenia, Mania, Acute psychotic disorders.
- Organic disorders—Delirium, Dementia and other organic psychosis.
- Withdrawal from alcohol or other drugs.
- Intoxication with alcohol, cannabinoids, amphetamines.
- Catatonic excitement.
- Acute stress reaction.
- Delirium due to any cause.
- Personality disorders.

Nursing Management

Following nursing principles should be followed for excited patients:

- Patients should be attended immediately. The most effective approach is to talk to the patient.
- Take care of your safety, do not approach alone.
- Keep optimal distance from patient and do not close the door of the consulting room.
- Ensure availability of adequate staff members for any emergency situation like physical restrain.
- Do not challenge or confront a violent patient.
- Verbal communication should be concise, concrete and unambiguous. Often the patients feel relieved to have someone to talk with; who he feels is going to help him.
- Benzodiazepines and anti psychotics are used most often for tranquilization.
- Restraint should be used as last resort and if necessary, should always be done in humane way.
- Hospitalization may be necessary to prevent violence, and for detailed assessment of the patient.

SUICIDE

Suicide: Suicide is a conscious act of killing oneself intentionally.

Attempted suicide: Attempted suicide refers to non-fatal suicidal behavior. Instead terms such as parasuicide or deliberate self harm (DSH) are preferred to represent acts deliberately undertaken by a person, which is not intended to result in fatal outcome.

Incidence: Rate of suicide is around 10 per 100,000 population , attempted suicides are estimated to be 10 to 20 times higher. 10% of those who attempt suicide subsequently commit suicide within 10 years.

Assessment of suicidal ideation: During examination always try to find out the thoughts of doing harm to himself, patient's intention, plan of executing suicidal thoughts, his current problems and psychiatric history.

Patient's family support system and risk for suicide in future should also be assessed (see Tables 26.1 and 26.2).

Nursing Management

- In emergency situations, when the patient is admitted following an attempt the priority is to stabilize the physical condition.
- Give an opportunity to express his feelings by providing sympathetic approach.

Table 26.1: Risk factors for suicide (Male)

- Use of violent methods (Hanging, Fire arms)
- Increasing age, particularly after age of 45
- Widowed, divorced or separated, living alone, socially isolated and recently bereaved
- Family history of suicide
- Higher social class
- Professionals particularly physicians
- Retirement and unemployment
- Chronic physical illness
- Hopelessness, isolation
- Psychiatric disorders like depression, alcoholism, drug abuse, schizophrenia, and personality disorder
- Past suicidal behavior.

Table 26.2: Risk factor for attempted suicide

- Females
- Younger people
- Lower social class, deprived background
- Unemployment
- Psychiatric disorders like depression
- Psychological problems like–Poor problem solving skills, Impulsivity, Interpersonal relationship problems
- Physical disorders like–Physical health problem, premenstrual syndrome in females.

- A thorough psychiatric assessment should be done.
- When a patient is found to have suicidal ideas on routine psychiatric evaluation, the clinician should inquire about co morbid medical illness and use of medication, substance abuse etc.
- The decision to treat the patient as inpatient or outpatient will depend on the diagnosis, severity of depression and suicidal ideation.
- Patient's safety is a nursing priority. In case of hospitalization, precaution must be taken to avoid further attempts while in hospital. This includes closer observation, searching patient's belongings and removing any items, which can be used as a weapon to harm one self.
- In an acutely depressed and suicidal patient, ECT should be considered, as the antidepressant takes time to act.
- If the patient is being treated as an outpatient, the patient's family should be made to take the responsibility for close monitoring of the patient.
- Treatment of the underlying psychiatric disorder such as depression or schizophrenia should follow the general guidelines for the treatment of these disorders.
- Psychotherapy with emphasis on reducing the ongoing stressors, enlisting social support, building better coping strategies and alternatives to suicide are useful in some of the patients.
- Suicide prevention can be done by identifying and managing those at risk.
- Crisis intervention is essential for the person with interpersonal and marital problems. Crisis interventions include ventilation, abreaction, and resolving conflicts.

DELIRIUM

Delirium is an acute organic mental syndrome characterized by global cognitive impairment, confusion, disorientation, increased psychomotor activity, visual hallucinations and sympathetic over activity. Delirium is often reversible and the course is brief and rapidly fluctuating. Delirium is commonly seen in the medically ill and in patients in intensive care units. It can also occur as a psychoactive substance withdrawal phenomenon. Old age, brain damage, infection and head injury predispose to delirium (For causes see Chapter 16).

Nursing Management

- Asses the vital parameters and level of consciousness at regular interval.
- Immediate management consists of good nursing care, maintenance of fluid and electrolyte balance and other supportive measures.
- Physical restraint may be used, if the patient is agitated.
- Haloperidol is the drug of choice, in a dose of 5-10 mg IM stat, the injection may be

repeated after 30 minutes if there is no response.

- Benzodiazepines like diazepam (5-10 mg) or lorazepam (1-2 mg) orally or intramuscularly may be used for agitation.
- Delirium has been discussed in detail in Chapter 16.

OTHER EMERGENCIES

PANIC ATTACKS

Panic attacks are characterized by spontaneous, episodic and intense period of anxiety, usually lasting about 20-30 minutes, and occurring on an average twice a week. Patient often presents with palpitation, sweating, shaking, dizziness, shortness of breath, chest pain and fear of dying and fainting. Generalized anxiety, thyrotoxicosis, withdrawal state, phobias and cardiac condition like mitral valve prolapse are the important differential diagnosis.

Immediate management consists of benzodiazepines, such as alprazolam 0.25 to 0.5 mg or lorazepam 1-2 mg, given orally 4 hourly or paroxetine 20-40 mg 2-3 times daily. Once the acute phase is over, long term management with anxiolytics and antidepressant, and or behavior therapy should be planned. A nursing care plan for increased anxiety and fear can be used for management.

INTOXICATION

Intoxication is defined as maladaptive behavior such as belligerence, impaired judgment and impairment social or occupational functioning, associated with recent psychoactive substance ingestion.

Common psychotropic substances involved include alcohol, cannabinoids, amphetamines, barbiturates, and opioids.

Management consists of nursing care, maintaining vital signs and supportive treatment. If patient is violent, appropriate treatment should be given. Drug treatment depends on the substance taken and the patient's clinical needs. If tranquilization is needed, benzodiazepines are preferred. However, medication should preferably be avoided.

STUPOR

Stupor is characterized by immobility and absence of response to stimuli without loss of consciousness. The patient is conscious but non-responsive to the environment. There is total lack of self-care with retention of urine and stool and the patient often stops oral intake. These patients are at special risk and may starve to death.

Important causes are catatonic schizophrenia, retarded depression, conversion disorder and organic conditions like head injuries, tumors of third ventricals etc.

Management consists of identifying the cause and treating it. Maintenance of nutrition and good nursing care are the essential components of treatment. ECT is preferred in depressive and catatonic stupor.

MANAGMENT OF THE SOCIAL AND PERSONAL CRISIS

Common crisis or emergency situations in personal or social areas include rape, marital crisis and acute grief reaction. Such problems are becoming increasingly common in emergency practice. The evaluation follows the usual format as described earlier. Further management should follow the guideline mentioned below:

RAPE

Rape is life threatening experience and may have life long psychological sequels. Therefore, rape victims need immediate and appropriate therapeutic intervention. The patient should be reassured and provided support. The patient should be encouraged to vent out her feelings. Appropriate medical, gynecological and police help should be provided. Management should include crisis intervention psychotherapy. Main objective is to minimize the psychological trauma of the assault on the victim. The patients often needs sedation, which may be given with benzodiazepines. Subsequently psychiatric referral may be indicated.

MARITAL CRISIS

Marital crisis refers to a serious conflict which may involve either or both the partners. Cause may include discovery of an extramarital affair, sexual problems in marriage, financial problems or disagreements about child rearing. One should always look for domestic violence. Both the members should be interviewed separately as well as jointly. If any one of them is suffering from psychiatric illness, it should be managed appropriately. The management is aimed at restructuring the relationship and improving communication.

ACUTE GRIEF REACTION

The characteristic feeling precipitated by the death of a loved one or following any other significant loss is called grief. Grief is usually a self limiting process but sometimes it is abnormal, and the patient may show severe depressive symptoms, psychotic features, agitation, suicidal impulses, and alcohol or drug abuse. The patient should be encouraged to express his/her feeling about the deceased, and reassured that the symptoms are normal and would remit with time. If any severe disturbance is noted, sedatives may be prescribed and appropriate psychiatric help should be sought.

One should never overlook patients who do not express significant grief, these patients should always be encouraged to express their emotions and be explored, why it is difficult for them to do so.

KEY POINTS

- Completed suicides are more common in men where as attempted suicides are common in women.
- Excited and violent patients are most common among psychiatric emergencies.
- Suicide is a common cause of death in psychiatric patients.
- Suicide rate in India is approximately 10 per lakh per year.
- Attempted suicides are 10-20 times more than actual suicides.
- Depression is the most common cause of suicide.
- In emergency situations, when the patient is admitted following an attempt through the emergency room, the priority is to stabilize the physical condition. Give an opportunity to express his feelings by providing sympathetic approach to the patient.
- A thorough psychiatric assessment should be done.
- In an acutely depressed and suicidal patient, ECT should be considered, as the antidepressant takes time to act.
- Patients should be attended immediately. The most effective approach is to talk to the patient. Take care of your safety, do not approach alone.
- Assessment, reassurance, sedation and restraint if necessary, are important steps in management of a violent patient.

- Alcohol is the most commonly linked drug to violence.
- Stupor is characterized by immobility and absence of response to stimuli without loss of consciousness. The patient is conscious but non-responsive to the environment.
- Organic stupor may occur due to head injury, tumors of basal ganglia, limbic system and frontal lobes, metabolic disorders.
- Functional stupor may occur due to schizophrenia, depression and mania.

27 Psychosocial Rehabilitation

Psychosocial rehabilitation refers to rehabilitation of chronically mentally ill patients. Rehabilitation is the process of enabling an impaired person to renew old skills or to acquire new skills, to prepare him to reintegrate in the society in a useful manner.

AIMS

Psychosocial rehabilitation includes various areas and activities. Rehabilitation in simple words means restoring the sick person to his optimal level of functioning. Following are the aims of rehabilitation:

- To reduce disability and improve functioning of the chronically mentally ill.
- To prepare him to join the mainstream of the society to which he belongs.
- Early identification of the patient and implementation of appropriate pharmacotherapy and non-pharmacological therapies at the earliest.

Early identification and early intervention prevent chronicity and hence reduce disability and improve the prospect of rehabilitation.

In rehabilitation work, three terms are frequently used often interchangeably. These are impairment, disability and handicap.

- **Impairment** refers to loss of function.
- **Disability** refers to loss of ability to perform a function because of a disorder.
- **Handicap** refers to the disadvantage and limitations conferred on the person with impairment and disability by the society.

Thus, impairment is important from an individual patient's perspective, disability is in the context of a medical perspective whereas handicap is a concern of the society.

REHABILITATIVE TEAM

Any rehabilitation work involves multidisciplinary team with all three participants i.e. the patient, mental health professionals and the society. The key members of the mental health professional team involved in psychosocial rehabilitation are the psychiatrist as the team leader and other such as psychiatric social workers, clinical psychologists, psychiatric and general nurses, occupational therapist and various types of vocational instructors. The role of psychiatric nurse in particular has great importance because of her long association with patients admitted in ward. A psychiatric nurse can motivate patients for participation in different rehabilitative programes as per their need.

To deliver rehabilitation services effectively and to confer maximum benefit on the patients, all these workers and agencies have to work harmoniously and in unison.

ASSESSMENT OF DISABILITIES

The assessment of patients for psychosocial rehabilitation is an important part of the process of rehabilitation. It includes assessment of:

- Impairments due to symptoms of delusions, hallucinations, thought disorders and distorted reality testing.

- Social problems such as homelessness, hostile family environment, social stigma and lack of sense of belonging.
- Disturbed level of social and vocational skills, unemployment or functioning of the patients.
- Personal and psychological needs of the patients.

Chronically mental ill patients have needs in various domains; the most prominent of them are needs relating to food, shelter, money, work, social and inter-personal relationship and utilization of time. The key members of team comprising mental health professionals contribute by assessing the patient's need and skills, the occupational therapist assesses domestic skills and so on. Depending on the assessment, the plan of activities for psychosocial rehabilitation is formulated and steps to implement it are also taken.

LEVEL OF INTERVENTIONS

A successful psychosocial rehabilitation programme is multidisciplinary and multimodal. Few specific level of interventions of rehabilitation depending upon need of individual patients and his family are given below:

Individual level	*Family level*	*Community level*
1. Pharmacotherapy	1. Psychoeducation	1. Day care centre
2. Supportive therapy	2. Family therapy	2. Half way home
3. Functional assessment		3. Institutionalized care
4. Social skill training		

1. Pharmacotherapy

Emphasis on pharmacotherapy assumes more significance in the light of research evidence that vigorous early intervention in psychosis improves rehabilitation prospects of the patients. The aim of the pharmacotherapy is to bring relief to the patient with regard to the florid psychotic symptoms and social and family disruption caused because of such symptoms. Pharmacotherapy also plays significant part in the relapse prevention. Drug non-compliance is a major issue in chronic mental disorders. If patients do not take prescribed medicines as directed, then disability and chronicity increase. Because of her close proximity with patients psychiatric nurse can motivate them to take medicines regularly as prescribed by consultant. She can also observe early signs of side effects of drug if any and report to the doctor.

2. Supportive Therapy

Supportive therapy is most widely accepted and practiced form of individual therapy for the mentally sick patients during course of rehabilitation. This therapy mainly includes:

- To educate the patient about mental illness, the role of prescribed medicines and importance of recognizing early signs of relapse. The net effect will lead to improved medication compliance and symptom control.
- The strategies to reduce the distress experienced by the patients in the course of everyday life problems enhance the patient sense of hope, educate him about the association of symptoms with stress and coping skills.
- To understand the psychological and social development and their illness experiences so as to inculcate in them a sense of themselves and foster recognition.

Individual supportive therapy is best meant for those patients, who have achieved a stable remission, demonstrated a solid therapeutic alliance. The major aim is to convey that therapist can be trusted, wants to understand the patient and has faith in the patient's potential as a human being.

3. Functional Assessment

Functional assessment of the patient, especially in the early phases of the illness, helps to plan the treatment process and allow professionals to prepare target interventions according to patient's specific needs. In chronic psychiatric conditions number of deficits including cognitive deficits, in turn, impair the ability to function independently. Therefore, functional assessment should include an evaluation of patient's performance in other areas especially self-care and social adjustment. A wide range of tools are available for assessment of these areas. After assessment of patient's day to day functional skills and abilities or deficits in self care, work and leisure, clinician can choose intervention that will enable the patient to achieve the highest level of functioning in the desired activity. This may include not only skill building, but also environmental support for those who may require it.

4. Social Skill Training (SST)

Impairment in social functioning is almost characteristic of schizophrenia. It limits patient's social opportunity with resulting rejection and isolation.

Social skills are defined as those interpersonal behaviors which are necessary for survival in community and social situations. The type of skills include communication skills, assertiveness skills, problem solving skills, skills related to specific activities, daily living etc. Social Skill Training (SST) is highly structured psychosocial intervention based on behavioral and learning principles and emphasizes modeling, role playing and social repertories, such as going for a job interview, maintaining eye contact and initiating communication etc. Patients are first taught the elements and then gradually learn how to perform them smoothly in sequence. In addition to modeling and role play, structured problem solving skills are employed to enable the patient to function in real life situations.

Studies demonstrate that effects of SST are maintained over 6-12 months and help in reducing the relapse rate when combined with adequate pharmacotherapy. Further maintenance of social skill training may require booster sessions. Social skills can be implemented in both individual and group setting with patients and their families. The patients, who are selected for SST have moderate to severe deficits in social functioning and SST is not needed for the better functioning patients.

Table 22.1: Common ingredients of family intervention programme

1. Involvement of the family early in treatment process.
2. Education about psychiatric disorders
   - Etiology
   - Variation in prognosis
   - Available treatment programme
   - The vulnerability stress model
   - Recommendations for coping with the disorder.
3. Communication Training
   - Improving communication in general
   - Improving ways of providing negative and positive feedback with in the family.
4. Problem Solving Training
   - Management of day to day problems and hassles
   - Management of discrete stressful life events
   - Generalized problem solving skills.
5. Crisis intervention.

Table 22.2: Do's & don'ts of family therapy

While aiming at Psychological rehabilitation of patient, the family should	- Not do anything which can cause relapse. - Not make the patient feel that he is less loved/cared/respected. - Do all the necessary help to make him to accept himself and develop positive attitude toward himself or others.
While aiming at social rehabilitation of patient, the family should	- Provide a status to the patient. - Accept that he is capable of earning a status to the family. - Strive for achieving good relationship. - Not have any unrealistic expectation from him.

INTERVENTIONS AT LEVEL OF FAMILY

5. Psychoeducational Family Therapy

The need to maintain the patient in community at an optimal level of functioning necessitates viewing the family as an important resource in the overall management. There is now convincing evidence that "Family intervention" is more effective than "routine care". Family interventions play an important role in improving medication compliance, delaying relapses and improving social functioning than individual therapies. The family interventions focus on two major areas:

1. Symptom reduction.
2. Family reaction to illness.

If the patient is in regular contact with family members, it is advisable to engage these relatives in the patient's care. Most studies have indicated that a program which covers a 9-12-month period following hospital discharge is acceptable to both patient and their relatives. Table 27.1 presents the essential components found useful in such a program and Table 27.2 exhibits do's and don'ts of family therapy.

INTERVENTIONS AT COMMUNITY LEVEL

In addition to individual and family focused interventions, management of treated chronic psychiatric conditions also demands effective development and utilization of community resources. Community based care encompasses a variety of services including day care and residential care.

6. Day Care Centre

It refers to comprehensive and multidisciplinary ambulatory treatment programs that include psychiatric, psychosocial and pre-vocational treatment modalities designed for patients with severe mental illness. Day care centre may be located in a psychiatric hospital, a general hospital, community health centre or be free standing. Usually the former provide for more "acute" short term care, while the latter is more supportive, long term management and for maintenance oriented services for chronic patient.

Day care facilities usually provide full range of medical and psychosocial treatment including family interventions. However, emphasis is on providing a social setting that is not merely concerned with reduction of disability, but also concern with social disadvantage of handicap. "Work" has traditionally been a source of social integration. Work in a day care setting is used to refer to any structured, purposeful and productive activity.

A group of patients may not be able to pursue any work related activity. Such patients still benefit from a setting where they can be engaged in social, leisure and recreational activities. They can be taught basic self-help skills or domestic living skills and provided a place to meet and be with people. Patients with chronic schizophrenia do better in a non-instructive, non-demanding social environment with more objects, focussed activity such as occupational therapy. Thus in Day Care setting, nurses have the tough task of balancing adequate work oriented care and non-threatening social environment.

7. Residential Care

This is the most important psychosocial intervention, which aims at improving functional disabilities by providing affordable and supportive housing. It has been divided into two categories:

1. Short term care.
2. Long term care.

Transitional half way homes (short term care): It is an intermediary point between leaving the hospital and returning to the family. It provides short term stay with 24 hours daily supervision for those patients who in due course of time would move to permanent housing in the community. In half way homes, during stay, the patients are not only are imparted training in living skills and interpersonal relationship, but family members are also encouraged to visit periodically and on weekends to take them out. Such centres cater mainly to mild to moderately ill and not to severely disabled for whom long term care in the form of custodial care unit are needed.

Institutional care (Long term care): Long term group residence are meant for long term stay with 24 hour daily supervision for those patients, who are unable to move out to permanent housing in the community from transitional half way homes.

STATUS OF REHABILITATION IN INDIA

Rehabilitation in India is still in its infancy. Although rehabilitation sub program for psychiatric patients in the community was envisaged in National Mental Health Programme. Yet because of variety of reasons it could not be implemented. At government level, policy makers have been unable to devote serious attention to the development of rehabilitation services for the chronic mentally ill, primarily due to economic constraints. To make the spectrum of rehabilitation service a reality in India, mental health professionals will have to actively collaborate with non-governmental sector. It is essential that we pool our expertise and knowledge base, so that we make the optimal use of the available resources. Studies have documented that distress and burden of caring for an ill relative are high and disruptive to daily routines.

Looking at the severity of problem, there is urgent need for more day care centres that can provide the much needed respite for the family as well as make the individual patients feel less stigmatized and more valued. Day care centre are the corner stones of community care. Similarly vocational training in such centre can help the patient to relearn or retain marketable skills. India being a prominently agricultural nation will always have a need for unskilled and semiskilled labor. A class of patients can surely be utilized in these services. Mobilization of government and private sector in this regard is the need of the hour.

KEY POINTS

- Rehabilitation is the process of enabling an impaired person to renew old skills or to acquire new skills, to prepare him to reintegrate in the society in a useful manner.
- Aim of Psychosocial rehabilitation includes early identification and early intervention to prevent chronicity and disability.
- Impairment is loss of normal functioning at organ level.
- Disability is disturbance due to impairment in performing normal functions.
- Handicap refers to disadvantages suffered by an individual as a result of impairments and disabilities.
- Psychosocial rehabilitation programme has multidisciplinary and multimodal approach, which have specific levels of interventions of rehabilitation, depending upon need of individual patients and his family.
- Rehabilitative intervention at individual level includes Pharmacotherapy, Supportive therapy, Functional assessment and Social skill training.
- Day care centre acts as a place of transition or link between the hospital and the community. Vocational training, occupational therapy, and social skills training including assertiveness training are being carried out from day care centres.

- Psychoeducation heips in removing misconception about mental disorders and their management, create awareness of side effects of drug and how to deal with day to day problems in life to reduces stress as well as distress.
- Intervention at community level demands effective development and utilization of community resources which include day care and residential care centre.
- Social skills are defined as those interpersonal behaviors which are not only necessary for mere survival in community but also in those demanding social situations which facilitate interpersonal relations and one's own social goes.
- Types of social skills include communication skills, assertiveness skills, problem solving skills, skills related to specific activities daily living etc.
- The role of psychiatric nurse in particular has great importance because of her long association with patients admitted in ward. A psychiatric nurse can motivate patients for participation in different rehabilitative programes as per their need.

28 Community Mental Health Services: Role of Nurse

Community mental health services include all those mental health activities in the community, which focus on the total population of defined geographical area rather than individual patient. Community mental health services mainly emphasize on organized programmes for the promotion of mental health, the prevention and treatment of mental disorders, and the rehabilitation of former psychiatric patients to meet all mental health service needs of the community. Other terms used for Community mental health services are community psychiatry, preventive psychiatry, outreach psychiatry, public health psychiatry. It has been called the "third psychiatric revolution" (the first being the age of enlightenment following the middle ages and the second being the development of psychoanalysis).

Community mental health nursing is the application of nursing knowledge in preventing, promoting and maintaining mental health of people.

DEVELOPMENT OF COMMUNITY HEALTH

In 1963, the US Congress passed the Community Mental Health Centers Act, which provided funds for the construction of Community Mental Health Centre (CMHC) with specified catchment areas. Each CMHC must provide five basic psychiatric services: impairment care, emergency services, community consultation, day care (including partial hospitalization programmes, half way houses, after care services, and a broad range of outpatient services), and research and education.

Community Mental Health Team

The community mental health team includes psychiatrists (including child psychiatrist), clinical psychologist, psychiatric social workers, psychiatric nurses, necessary administrative helps and clerical staff, and occupational and recreational therapist for inpatient and partial hospitalization programmes. Links to welfare workers, clergy, family agencies, schools and other human services groups are also maintained.

Long Term Care

Community Mental Health Programmes encourage continuity of care. This continuity of care enables a single clinician to follow a given patient through emergency services, hospitalization, partial hospitalization as a transition to the community, and outpatient treatment as follow-up. It also provides an exchange of information and team responsibility for the patient when different therapists treat the patient in different settings.

Community Participation

The community should participate in decisions about its mental health care needs and programmes, instead of having them solely defined by professionals. Mental health services are sensitive to the needs of those served if the public is actively involved.

PREVENTION IN PSYCHIATRY

The prevention for psychiatric disorders follow the same principles as in case of other disorders and has been divided into primary, secondary and tertiary prevention. The goal of preventive efforts is to decrease the onset (incidence), duration (prevalence), and residual disability of mental disorders.

Primary Prevention

The goal of primary prevention is to prevent the onset of a disease or disorder thereby reducing its incidence. This goal is accomplished by eliminating etiological factors, strengthening host resistance, or interfering with the mode of disease transmission.

The aim of primary prevention is to help the individual to cope with mental health problems (include mental health education programmes for parent training in child development and alcohol and drug education programs, to aim at competence building, development and utilization of social support systems to reduce the effects of stress on persons at high risk), anticipatory guidance programs to assist people in preparing for expected stressful situations and crisis intervention following the occurrence of stressful life events such as bereavement, marital separation and divorce, individual traumas or group disasters.

Community mental health nurse has a significant role in primary prevention. She has a significant role in pre and post natal care, which can help in reduction in mental retardation and other organic mental disorders. Similarly she can guide children and adolescents for their mental health and drug addiction problems. She can also be part of various mental health education programes of vulnerable groups, in which she can act as educator, trainer and group leader.

Secondary Prevention

Secondary prevention is defined as early identification and prompt treatment of an illness or disorder with the goal of reducing the prevalence. By providing rapid treatment of emerging mental disorders in the social milieu of the patient's home community with the expectation that he can improve, a clinician can facilitate a patient's recovery.

Secondary prevention is possible with services including emergency services, outpatient clinics, day treatment programmes and community based units. The emphasis is on minimizing the duration of illness. In case a patient requires medication then a psychiatrists should be consulted immediately. Nurse can also help in early detection and prompt treatment of mental health problems among high risk individuals such as persons in crisis situations, high school children, recently divorced and widowed, retired persons etc. Community mental health nurse could be an instrumental person in management of crisis. Crisis intervention is a process by which an individual is helped to cope with a crisis in his or her life situation, so as to bring his level of functioning to that of previous level.

Tertiary Prevention

The goal of tertiary prevention is to reduce the prevalence of residual defect or disability due to illness or disorder. In the case of psychiatric conditions, tertiary prevention involves rehabilitative efforts to enable those who have a chronic mental illness to reach the highest level of functioning. The disabilities associated with chronic mental illness represent major social, economic and public health problems.

The broad range of services necessary for community based tertiary prevention include comprehensive emergency services; acute inpatient facilities; partial hospitalization; outpatient programmes that provide medication monitoring;

psychosocial, individual, group and family therapies; psychosocial peer and family support organization; to support agencies and provide aggressive outreach services to patients reluctant to keep in contact with the treatment system; and a variety of social and vocational rehabilitation programs.

Mental Health in India–At a Glance

Existing mental health problems and services in India.

Problems

- 1% of population suffer from severe mental disorders like schizophrenia and other psychosis (10-12 million).
- About 10% of population suffer from minor mental disorders like anxiety, neurotic disorders etc. (100 million).
- 20-30% of patients in general clinical setting are suffering from an underlying psychiatric disorder.
- Suicide rate in India is about 10 per lakh population.
- About 1-2% of total children have some underlying psychiatric problem.
- About 0.5-1.0% of all children have mental retardation.

Resources

- About 25000 beds in 37 mental hospitals and 2000 to 3000 psychiatric beds in general and teaching hospitals.
- First mental hospital was built in Bombay (now Mumbai).
- In India with population of one billion, there is one psychiatric bed per 30000 population.
- 3500-4000 qualified psychiatrists, 800-1000 clinical psychologists and 400-500 psychiatric social workers available to look after these problems (one psychiatrist per 3-4 lakh population).

ROLE OF NURSE IN COMMUNITY MENTAL HEALTH

Community Mental Health Nursing is the application of knowledge of psychiatric nursing in preventing, promoting and maintaining mental health of the people, to help in early diagnosis and care and to rehabilitate the patients after mental illness.

In community living, the individual may go through stressful situations. He/she may or may not be able to cope with stress and adjustment take places. Sometime this stress leads to mental illness. The role of nurse in community setting can be viewed from different angles. Nurse can help in attaining the goal of community mental health being the part of multidisciplinary approach. Nurse play a pivotal role in primary, secondary and tertiary prevention of mental illness.

Primary Prevention

Primary prevention means lowering the rate of new cases of mental disorders in a population by counteracting forces which may produce illness, like providing health education to vulnerable groups of teenagers, homeless families. The emphasis in primary prevention is mainly on health development and effective coping abilities of an individual. Like other diseases, number of factors play an important role in etiology of mental disorders. Such factors may be:

1. Biological and physical factors.
2. Psychosocial factors.
3. Sociocultural factors.

Biological and Physical Factors

The community health has a significant role especially in prenatal and postnatal care. It help in reduction of mental retardation and organic mental disorders. By advising them for regular antenatal check up, on nutrition, vaccination, avoidance of the use of drugs and alcohol, repeated X-rays, prevention of repeated abortions, genetic counselling etc. she can help in prevention of disorders like mental retardation, mongolism, AIDS and malnutrition. A childless couple should be guided for the investigation for adoption for their mental health.

Psychosocial Factors

The individual needs to learn all those competencies by which he/she can cope with crisis situations. Nurse can help the target group in achieving physical, intellectual, emotional and social competencies to cope with difficult and stressful situations and keep them mentally healthy. Such preparations of individuals help them to cope with changes such as adolescence, marriage, pregnancy, childbirth, family planning, marriage of children and old age.

Similarly mental health education among masses and vulnerable groups through public education programme, TV programme, radio talks, articles, health exhibitions also help in individual coping to stress.

Sociocultural Factors

Strengthening of social support system for risk group population like widows, adolescents, primi mother, death of spouse, divorcee, victim of earthquakes or bomb explosion is also a preventive strategy, for which the nurse's role is important. A nurse can arrange public education programme, training programme for parents and school teachers, street plays, exhibitions and group meetings of specific groups.

Secondary Prevention

The approach of the community mental health nursing in secondary prevention should be early detection and prompt intervention of high-risk individuals such as recently divorced or widowed, victims of earth quake, high school dropouts, and retirement. In these crisis situations, intervention helps the individual to recover fast, otherwise precipitation of crisis leads to anxiety, fear, guilt, shame and helplessness.

The community mental health nurse needs to identify the available outpatient and inpatient treatment within the community. Partial/short-term hospitalization like day-care centres can be utilized. Effort should be made to minimize the duration of sickness. If a patient requires drug, or physical therapy (ECT), the psychiatrist should be consulted immediately. Follow-up should be done to ensure the improvement or deterioration of the patient's mental and physical health. Crisis intervention must be considered a very significant aspect of secondary prevention.

Tertiary Prevention

The goal of tertiary prevention is to reduce the prevalence of long-term disabilities and problems due to mental disorders. Tertiary prevention includes prompt and intensive inpatient care, rehabilitation, after-care and reconciliation. Intensive inpatient care for emotional disorders will prevent it from becoming chronic. It will also enable the individual to return to his home or society as early as possible. Through the community mental health approach the following therapeutic services can be provided by the nurse:

1. **Treatment and follow-up:** The community mental health nurse needs to ensure the type of psychotropic drugs the patient is taking. She also needs to ensure maintenance of dose, supervision of safe intake of drugs, observation of side-effects, educating family members to observe for side-effects and report.
2. **Individual and family therapy:** The patient has to go back to his family. So it is very essential that the family is helped to meet the stress. Family support needs to be identified in helping the patient.
3. **Crisis intervention:** Crisis intervention deals with the present situation and resolution of the immediate issue. Early intervention in assisting the individual to manage the current situation promotes the best chance for a positive outcome. Once the anxiety level is reduced to a tolerable level, the individual can be assisted in defining the problem, determining available support, and setting realistic goals for resolution of the issue. The nurse is integral in providing support and returning control to the patient.
4. **Rehabilitative services:** Rehabilitation and after-care is an essential aspect for complete management of mentally disordered patients.

The patient needs to be rehabilitated and helped to become socially productive. They need to readjust themselves outside the hospital. They should be provided with 'safe and human' therapeutic housing. It may be required for patients who are recovering as for those with chronic diseases. Therapeutic housing may be supervised or unsupervised. His areas of interest can be explored and he can be helped to pick up a job. This support can be provided by members of the family and the community and mental health team.

Community facilities for mentally disordered patients after discharge from the hospital are described as follows:

A. **Day Hospital/Centres:** This facility is organized on a day-time basis. The patient receives a full range of treatment, services and returns home at the end of the day. The concept, introduced by D.E. Cameran in 1946, is now being used in rehabilitation and psychiatric care. A day hospital is staffed by trained psychiatric and other team members. In India, only a few day care centers are available for mentally ill, but comparatively better for mentally retarded. The family feels relief a for few hours in a day and develops coping energy for the rest of the time when the patient is at home. The patient develops discipline and routine.

B. **Half-way Home:** It is a transition facility for psychiatric patients who no longer need the full services of a hospital but are not yet ready for a completely independent living. They need supervision for medication and for carrying on domestic activities. If they are still in job, they will leave for the job and come back to this half-way house. Medical facilities are regularly provided.

C. **Group Homes:** These homes may belong to hospital or rented by 15 to 20 mentally ill recovering patients. These ex-patients stay together, meet their financial commitments and live in a socicty like other members. They try to provide moral, emotional and social support to each other. If one of the members is leading towards relapse, others try to help him by providing support.

D. **Foster Homes:** It is a home in which a patient recovering from a mental disorder is placed in voluntary family by a social agency for family care. The family is paid by the agency. Placement may be temporary or permanent. The patient gets a home-like environment.

E. **Sheltered Workshop:** It is a work-oriented rehabilitation facility with a controlled working environment to fulfill the individual's vocational goals. In these workshops ex-long-term mentally ill patients can utilize their experience and abilities by relearning. This helps the patient to make progress towards a normal living and economic independence.

F. **Self-Help Groups:** Self-help groups in the community will help the individual as well as members of the family. Alcoholic anonymous groups, drug addiction groups, groups of patients with mental retardation are a few of the examples.

Thus community mental health nursing provides comprehensive, continuous care to the people. The aim is to reduce the number of mentally ill patients through primary prevention; early diagnosis and limiting the disability; through secondary prevention and rehabilitation, through use of community facilities by tertiary prevention.

The community mental health nurse applies her knowledge of the nursing process in assessment, planning, implementation intervention and evaluation to provide comprehensive care to patients.

NATIONAL MENTAL HEALTH PROGRAMME (1982)

According to WHO "Health" is defined as a positive state of physical, mental and social well-being, not merely absence of illness. Mental health is thus an integral component of total health. Availability of psychiatric services to the rural population (which consists of three-fourth of our population) still remains extremely inadequate. To find a solution of these problems, an expert group was formed in 1980. The final draft was submitted to the Central Council of Health and Family Welfare on August 18-20 1982, which recommended its implementation. The NMHP appeared almost simultaneously with the National Health Policy (1993).

Objectives of National Mental Health Programme

- To ensure availability and accessibility of minimum mental health care for all in the foreseeable future, particularly to the most vulnerable and under priviledged sections of population.
- To encourage application of mental health knowledge in general health care and in social development.
- To promote community participation in the mental health service development and to stimulate efforts towards self help in the community.

Aims

- Integration of the mental health care service with the existing general health services.
- To utilize the existing infra structure of health services and also to deliver the minimum mental health care service.
- To provide appropriate task oriented training to the existing health staff.
- To link mental health services with the existing community development programme.

Components

1. *Treatment:* The treatment programme has been planned keeping the primary health care (PHC) as the sheet anchor. At the same time, it consists of the creation of an appropriate referral system at various levels. As per NMHP mental health care is to be provided at different levels e.g. PHC at village level, District hospital, Psychiatric unit of medical colleges.
2. *Rehabilitation:* Rehabilitation of psychiatric patients will be facilitated greatly by maintenance treatment of epileptics and psychotics at community level.
3. *Prevention:* This component of the service programme will be community based with only a united involvement of the health service personnel and community leaders.

KEY POINTS

- Community psychiatry is a branch of psychiatry that develops and maintains organized programs for the promotion of mental health, the prevention and treatment of mental disorders, and the rehabilitation of former psychiatric patients.
- National mental health program (NMHP) of India was launched in 1982.
- Objectives of NMHP were: (i) To ensure availability and accessibility of minimum mental health care for all in the foreseeable future (ii) To encourage application of mental health knowledge in general health care and in social development (iii) To promote community participation in the mental health service.

- Primary prevention in psychiatry includes lowering the rate of new cases of mental disorders in population by modification of biological, psychological and social factors. Primary prevention includes mental health education programmes, mobilization of social support system and crisis intervention services.
- Secondary prevention aims at early detection and immediate treatment of maladaptive behavior in individual, family and society with the goal of reducing the prevalence.
- Secondary prevention is most effective type of prevention in psychiatry.
- Tertiary prevention aims at reducing the prevalence of residual defect or disability due to illness or disorder and involves rehabilitative efforts to enable those who have a chronic mental illness to reach the highest level of functioning feasible. The disabilities associated with chronic mental illness represent major social, economic and public health problems.

Appendices

APPENDIX-A

List of categories classified in International Classification of Disease-10 (ICD-10) of World Health Organization (F00-F99)

F0	Organic, including symptomatic, mental disorders	
F00	Dementia in Alzheimer's Disease	
	F00.0	Dementia in Alzheimer's Disease, with early onset
	F00.1	Dementia in Alzheimer's Disease, with late onset
	F00.2	Dementia in Alzheimer's disease, atypical or mixed type
	F00.9	Unspecified
F01	Vascular Dementia	
	F01.0	Vascular dementia of acute onset
	F01.1	Multi-infarct (predominantly cortical) vascular dementia
	F01.2	Subcortical vascular dementia
	F01.3	Mixed cortical and subcortical vascular dementia
	F01.8	Other
	F01.9	Unspecified
F02	Dementia in diseases classified elsewhere	
	F02.0	Dementia in Pick's disease
	F02.1	Dementia in Creutzfeldt-Jakob disease
	F02.2	Dementia in Huntington's disease
	F02.3	Dementia in Parkinson's disease
	F02.4	Dementia in HIV infection
	F02.8	Dementia in other diseases classified elsewhere
F03	Dementia, unspecified	
F04	Organic amnesic syndrome, other than induced by alcohol or drugs	
F05	Delirium, other than induced by alcohol or drugs	
	F05.0	Delirium, not superimposed on dementia
	F05.1	Delirium, superimposed on dementia
	F05.8	Other delirium
	F05.9	Delirium, unspecified
F06	Other mental disorders, due to brain disease, damage or dysfunction or to physical disease, including hormonal disturbances	
	F06.0	Organic hallucinations
	F06.1	Organic catatonic disorder
	F06.2	Organic delusional or schizophrenia-like disorder

Contd.

Contd.

	F06.3	Organic affective disorder	
		.30 Organic manic disorder	
		.31 Organic bipolar disorder	
		.32 Organic depressive disorder	
	F06.4	Organic anxiety disorders	
	F06.5	Organic dissociative disorders	
	F06.6	Organic emotionally labile disorders	
	F06.7	Organic cognative disorders	
	F06.8	Other	
	F06.9	Unspecified	
F07	Personality and behavioral disorders due to brain disease, damage or dysfunction		
	F07.0	Organic personality disorder	
	F07.1	Postencephalitic syndrome	
	F07.2	Postconcussional syndrome	
	F07.8	Other	
	F07.9	Unspecified	
F09	Organic or symptomatic mental disorders, unspecified		
F1	**Mental and behavioral disorders due to psychoactive and other substances use**		
F10	Disorders resulting from use of alcohol		
F11	Disorders resulting from use of opioids		
F12	Disorders resulting from use of cannabinoids		
F13	Disorders resulting from use of sedatives or hypnotics		
F14	Disorders resulting from use of cocaine		
F15	Disorders resulting from use of other stimulants		
F16	Disorders resulting from use of hallucinogens		
F17	Disorders resulting from use of tobacco		
F18	Disorders resulting from use of volatile solvents		
F19	Disorders resulting from multiple drug use and use of other and identified substances		
	4th and 5th character codes for specifying the clinical condition		
Flx.0	Acute intoxication		
	.00 uncomplicated		
	.01 with trauma or other bodily injury		
	.02 with other medical complication		
	.03 with delirium		
	.04 with perceptual distortions		
	.05 with coma		
	.06 with convulsions		
Flx.1	Harmful use		
Flx.2	Dependence syndrome		
	.20 currently abstinent		
	.21 currently abstinent, but in a protected environment		
	.22 currently or clinically supervised maintenance regime		
	.23 currently using the drug		
	.24 continuous use		
	.25 episodic use		

Contd.

Contd.

Flx.3	Withdrawal state .30 uncomplicated .31 with convulsions
Flx.4	Withdrawal state with delirium .40 without convulsions .41 with convulsions
Flx.5	Psychotic disorder .50 Schizophrenia like .51 predominantly delusional .52 predominantly hallucinatory .53 predominantly polymorphic .54 predominantly depressive symptoms .55 predominantly manic symptoms .56 mixed
Flx.6	Alcohol or drug induced amnesic syndrome
Flx.7	Alcohol or drug induced residual and late onset psychotic disorder .70 flashbacks .71 personality or behavior disorder .72 affective state .73 dementia .74 other persisting cognitive impairment .75 late onset psychotic disorder
Flx.8	Other mental behavioral disorders induced by alcohol or drugs
Flx.9	Mental or behavioral disorder induced by alcohol or drugs, unspecified
F2	**Schizophrenia, schizotypal and delusional disorders**
F20	Schizophrenia F20.0 Paranoid schizophrenia F20.1 Hebephrenic schizophrenia F20.2 Catatonic schizophrenia F20.3 Undifferentiated schizophrenia F20.4 Post-schizophrenic depression F20.5 Residual schizophrenia F20.6 Simple schizophrenia F20.8 Other schizophrenia F20.9 Unspecified schizophrenia
F21	Schizotypal disorder
F22	Persistent delusional disorder F22.0 Delusional disorder F22.8 Other persistent delusional disorder F22.9 Unspecified
F23	Acute and transient psychotic disorder
F23.0	Acute polymorphic psychotic disorders (without symptoms of schizophrenia) .00 without associated acute stress .01 with associated acute stress
F23.1	Acute polymorphic psychotic disorders (with symptoms of schizophrenia) .10 without associated acute stress .11 with associated acute stress

Contd.

Contd.

F23.2	Acute schizophrenia like psychotic disorder	
	.20	without associated acute stress
	.21	with associated acute stress
F23.3	Other acute predominantly delusional psychotic disorder	
	.30	without associated acute stress
	.31	with associated acute stress
F23.8	Other acute and transient psychotic episode	
F23.9	Unspecified acute and transient psychotic episode	
F24	Induced delusional disorders (Follie and Deux)	
F25	Schizoaffective disorders	
	F25.0	Schizoaffective disorder, manic type
	F25.1	Schizoaffective disorder, depressive type
	F25.2	Schizoaffective disorder, mixed type
	F25.8	Other
	F25.9	Unspecified
F28	Other non-organic psychotic disorders	
F29	Non-organic psychosis, unspecified	
F3	**Mood (affective) disorders**	
F30	Manic episode	
F30.0	Hypomania	
F30.1	Mania without psychotic symptoms	
F30.2	Mania with psychotic symptoms	
	.20 psychotic symptoms mood congruent	
	.21 psychotic symptoms mood incongruent	
F30.8	Other	
F30.9	Unspecified	
F31	Bipolar affective disorder	
	F31.0	Current episode hypomania
	F31.1	Current episode manic without psychotic symptoms
	F31.2	Current episode manic with psychotic symptoms
		.20 psychotic symptoms mood congruent
		.21 psychotic symptoms mood incongruent
	F31.3	Current episode moderate or mild depression
		.30 moderate or mild depression without somatic symptoms
		.31 moderate or mild depression with somatic symptoms
	F31.4	Current episode severe depression without psychotic symptoms
	F31.5	Current episode severe depression with psychotic symptoms
		.50 psychotic symptoms mood congruent
		.51 psychotic symptoms mood incongruent
	F31.6	Current episode mixed
	F31.7	Currently remission
	F31.8	Other
	F31.9	Unspecified
F32	Depressive episode	
	F32.0	Mild severity
		.00 Mild severity without somatic symptoms
		.01 Mild severity with somatic symptoms

Contd.

Contd.

	F32.1	Moderate severity	
		.10 moderate severity without somatic symptoms	
		.11 moderate severity with somatic symptoms	
	F32.2	Severe depressive episode without psychotic symptoms	
	F32.3	Severe depressive episode with psychotic symptoms	
		.30 psychotic symptoms mood congruent	
		.31 psychotic symptoms mood incongruent	
	F32.8	Other	
	F32.9	Unspecified	
F33	Recurrent depressive disorder		
	F33.0	Current episode mild severity	
		.00 mild severity without somatic symptoms	
		.01 mild severity with somatic symptoms	
	F33.1	Current episode moderate severity	
		.10 moderate severity without somatic symptoms	
		.11 moderate severity with somatic symptoms	
	F33.2	Current episode severe without psychotic symptoms	
	F33.3	Current episode severe with psychotic symptoms	
		.30 psychotic symptoms mood congruent	
		.31 psychotic symptoms mood incongruent	
	F33.4	Currently in remission	
	F33.8	Other	
	F33.9	Unspecified	
F34	Persistent affective disorders		
	F34.0	Cyclothymia	
	F34.1	Dysthymia	
	F34.8	Other	
	F34.9	Unspecified	
F38	Other mood (affective) disorders		
	F38.0	Other single affective episode	
	F38.1	Other recurrent affective disorder	
	F38.8	Other	
F39	Affective disorders, unspecified		
F4	**Neurotic, stress-related and somatoform disorders**		
F40	Phobic disorders		
	F40.0	Agoraphobia	
		.00 agoraphobia without panic disorder	
		.01 agoraphobia with panic disorder	
	F40.1	Social phobia	
	F40.2	Specific (isolated) phobias	
	F40.8	Other	
	F40.9	Unspecified	
F41	Other anxiety disorders		
	F41.0	Panic disorders	
	F41.1	Generalized anxiety disorder	
	F41.2	Mixed anxiety and depressive disorder	
	F41.3	Other mixed anxiety disorder	

Contd.

Contd.

	F41.8	Other
	F41.9	Unspecified
F42	Obsessive compulsive disorder	
	F42.0	Predominantly obsessional thoughts or ruminations
	F42.1	Predominantly compulsive acts (obsessional rituals)
	F42.2	Mixed obsessional thoughts and acts
	F42.8	Other
	F42.9	Unspecified
F43	Reaction to severe stress and adjustment disorders	
	F43.0	Acute stress reaction
	F43.1	Post traumatic stress disorder
	F43.2	Adjustment disorder
		.20 brief depressive reaction
		.21 prolonged depressive reaction
		.22 mixed anxiety and depressive reactions
		.23 with predominant disturbance of other emotions
		.24 with predominant disturbance of conduct
		.25 with mixed disturbance of emotions and conduct
		.28 other specified
	F43.8	Other
	F43.9	Unspecified
F44	Dissociative (conversion) disorders	
	F44.0	Dissociative amnesia
	F44.1	Dissociative fugue
	F44.2	Dissociative stupor
	F44.3	Trance and possession disorders
	F44.4	Dissociative movement disorders
	F44.5	Dissociative convulsions
	F44.6	Dissociative anesthesia and sensory loss
	F44.7	Mixed dissociative and conversion disorders
	F44.8	Other
	F44.9	Unspecified
F45	Somatoform disorder	
	F45.0	Somatization disorder
	F45.1	Undifferentiated somatoform disorder
	F45.2	Hypochondriacal disorder
	F45.3	Somatoform autonomic dysfunction
		.30 the heart and cardiovascular system
		.31 the esophagus and stomach
		.32 the lower gastrointestinal tract
		.33 the respiratory system
		.34 the urogenital system
	F45.4	Persistent pain disorder
	F45.8	Other
	F45.9	Unspecified

Contd.

Contd.

F48	Other neurotic disorders	
	F48.0	Neurasthenia (Fatigue syndrome)
	F48.1	Depersonalization-derealization syndrome
	F48.8	Other
	F48.9	Unspecified
F5	**Behavioral syndromes and mental disorders associated with physiological dysfunction**	
F50	Eating disorders	
	F50.0	Anorexia nervosa
	F50.1	Bulimia nervosa
	F50.2	Normal weight bulimia
	F50.3	Overeating associated with other psychological disturbances
	F50.4	Vomiting associated with other psychological disturbances
	F50.8	Other
	F50.9	Unspecified
F51	Sleep disorders, due to emotional causes	
	F51.0	Insomnia, due to emotional causes
	F51.1	Hypersomnia, due to emotional causes
	F51.2	Disorder of the sleep wake schedule, due to emotional causes
	F51.3	Sleepwalking
	F51.4	Sleep terrors
	F51.5	Nightmares
	F51.8	Other
	F51.9	Unspecified
F52	Sexual dysfunction, not caused by organic disorder or disease	
	F52.0	Lack or loss of sexual desire
	F52.1	Sexual aversion and lack of sexual enjoyment
		.10 sexual aversion
		.11 lack of sexual enjoyment
	F52.2	Failure of genital response
	F52.3	Orgasmic dysfunction
	F52.4	Premature ejaculation
	F52.5	Vaginismus
	F52.6	Dyspareunia
	F52.7	Excessive sexual drive
	F52.8	Other
	F52.9	Unspecified
F53	Mental or behavioral disorders associated with puerperium, not classifiable elsewhere	
	F53.0	Mild mental disorder associated with the puerperium, not classifiable elsewhere
	F53.1	Severe mental disorders associated with the puerperium, not classifiable elsewhere
	F53.8	Other
	F53.9	Unspecified
F54	Psychological or behavioral factors associated with disorders or diseases classified elsewhere	
F59	Behavioral syndromes and mental disorders associated with physiological dysfunction, unspecified	
F6	**Disorders of adult personality and behavior**	
F60	Specific personality disorders	
	F60.0	Paranoid personality disorder

Contd.

Contd.

	F60.1	Schizoid personality disorder
	F60.2	Dissocial personality disorder
	F60.3	Emotionally unstable personality disorder
		.30 impulsive type
		.31 borderline type
	F60.4	Histrionic personality disorder
	F60.5	Anankastic (obsessive compulsive) personality disorder
	F60.6	Anxious (avoidant) personality disorder
	F60.7	Dependent personality disorder
	F60.8	Other
	F60.9	Unspecified
F61	Mixed and other personality disorder	
F62	Enduring personality changes, not attributable to gross brain damage or disease	
F62.0	Enduring personality change after catastrophic experience	
F62.1	Enduring personality change after psychiatric illness	
F62.8	Other	
F62.9	Unspecified	
F63	Habit and impulse disorder	
	F63.0	Pathological gambling
	F63.1	Pathological fire setting (pyromania)
	F63.2	Pathological stealing
	F63.3	Trichotillomania
	F63.8	Other
	F63.9	Unspecified
F64	Gender identity disorder	
	F64.0	Transsexualism
	F64.1	Dual role transvestism
	F64.2	Gender identity disorder or childhood
	F64.8	Other
	F64.9	Unspecified
F65	Disorders of sexual preferences	
	F65.0	Fetishism
	F65.1	Fetishistic transvestism
	F65.2	Exhibitionism
	F65.3	Voyeurism
	F65.4	Pedophilia
	F65.5	Sado-masochism
	F65.6	Multiple disorders of sexual preferences
	F65.8	Other
	F65.9	Unspecified
F66	Psychological and behavioral disorders associated with sexual development and orientation	
	F66.0	Sexual maturation disorder
	F66.1	Ego-dystonic sexual orientation
	F66.2	Sexual relationship disorders
	F66.8	Other
	F66.9	Unspecified

Contd.

Contd.

F68	Other disorders of adult personality and behavior		
	F68.0	Elaboration of physical symptoms for psychological reasons	
	F68.1	Intentional production or feigning of symptoms or disabilities, either physical or psychological (factitious disorder)	
	F68.8	Other specified disorders of adult personality and behavior	
F69	Disorder of adult personality and behavior, unspecified		
F7	**Mental disorders**		
F70	Mild mental retardation		
F71	Moderate mental retardation		
F72	Severe mental retardation		
F73	Profound mental retardation		
F78	Other mental retardation		
F79	Mental retardation, unspecified		
F8	**Disorders of psychological development**		
F80	Specific developmental disorders of speech and language		
	F80.0	Specific speech articulation disorder	
	F80.1	Expressive language disorder	
	F80.2	Receptive language disorder	
	F80.3	Acquired aphasia with epilepsy	
	F80.8	Other	
	F80.9	Unspecified	
F81	Specific developmental disorders of scholastic skills		
	F81.0	Specific reading disorder	
	F81.1	Specific spelling disorder	
	F81.2	Specific disorder of arithmetical disorder	
	F81.3	Mixed disorder of scholastic skills	
	F81.8	Other	
	F81.9	Unspecified	
F82	Specific developmental disorders of motor functions		
F83	Mixed specific developmental disorders		
F84	Pervasive developmental disorders		
	F84.0	Childhood autism	
	F84.1	Atypical autism	
	F84.2	Rett's syndrome	
	F84.3	Other childhood disintegrative disorders	
	F84.4	Overactive disorders associated with mental retardation and stereotyped movements	
	F84.5	Asperger's syndrome	
	F84.8	Other	
	F84.9	Unspecified	
F88	Other disorders of psychological developments		
F89	Disorders of psychological developmental, unspecified		
F9	**Behavioral and emotional disorders with onset usually occurring in childhood or adolescence (and mental disorder unspecified)**		
F90	Hyperkinetic disorders		
	F90.0	Disturbance of activity and attention	
	F90.1	Hyperkinetic conduct disorder	

Contd.

Contd.

	F90.8	Other
	F90.9	Unspecified
F91	Conduct disorder	
	F91.0	Conduct disorder confined to the family context
	F91.1	Unsocialized conduct disorder
	F91.2	Socialized conduct disorder
	F91.3	Oppositional defiant disorder
	F91.8	Other
	F91.9	Unspecified
F92	Mixed disorder of conduct and emotions	
	F92.0	Depressive conduct disorder
	F92.8	Other
	F92.9	Unspecified
F93	Emotional disorders with onset specific to childhood	
	F93.0	Separation anxiety disorder
	F93.1	Phobic disorder of childhood
	F93.2	Social sensitivity disorder
	F93.3	Sibling rivalry disorder
	F93.8	Other
	F93.9	Unspecified
F94	Disorders of social functioning with onset specific to childhood or adolescence	
	F94.0	Elective mutism
	F94.1	Reactive attachment disorder of childhood
	F94.2	Disinhibited attachment disorder of childhood
	F94.8	Other
	F94.9	Unspecified
F95	Tic disorder	
	F95.0	Transient tic disorder
	F95.1	Chronic motor or vocal tic disorder
	F95.2	Combined vocal and multiple motor tics (Tourett's Syndrome)
	F95.8	Other
	F95.9	Unspecified
F98	Other behavioral and emotional disorders with onset usually occurring during childhood or adolescence	
	F98.0	Enuresis
	F98.1	Encopresis
	F98.2	Feeding disorder of infancy or childhood
	F98.3	Pica
	F98.4	Stereotyped movement disorder
	F98.5	Stuttering
	F98.6	Cluttering
	F98.8	Other
	F98.9	Unspecified
F99	Mental disorders, unspecified	

APPENDIX-B

NANDA (North American Nursing Diagnosis Association) Approved Nursing Diagnoses

A

Activity intolerance
Activity intolerance, Risk for
Adjustment, Impaired
Airway clearance, Ineffective
Allergy response, Latex
Allergy response, Risk for latex
Anxiety
Anxiety, Death
Aspiration, Risk for
Attachment, Risk for impaired parent/infant/child
Autonomic dysreflexia
Autonomic dysreflexia, Risk for

B

Body image, Disturbed
Body temperature, Risk for imbalanced
Bowel incontinence
Breastfeeding, Effective
Breastfeeding, Ineffective
Breastfeeding, Interrupted
Breathing pattern, Ineffective

C

Cardiac output, Decreased
Caregiver role strain
Caregiver role strain, Risk for
Communication, Impaired verbal
Communication, Readiness for enhanced
Conflict, Decisional
Conflict, Parental role
Confusion, Acute
Confusion, Chronic
Constipation
Constipation, Perceived
Constipation, Risk for
Coping, Ineffective
Coping, Defensive
Coping, Readiness for enhanced
Coping, Ineffective community
Coping, Readiness for enhanced community
Coping, Compromised family
Coping, Readiness for enhanced family

D

Death syndrome, Risk for sudden
Denial, Ineffective
Dentition, Impaired
Development, Risk for delayed
Diarrhea
Disuse syndrome, Risk for
Diversional activity, Deficient

E

Energy field, Disturbed
Environmental interpretation syndrome, Impaired

F

Failure to thrive, Adult
Falls, Risk for
Family process, Interrupted
Family process, Readiness for enhanced
Fatigue
Fear
Fluid balance, Readiness for enhanced
Fluid volume, Deficient
Fluid volume, Excess
Fluid volume, Risk for deficient
Fluid volume, Risk for imbalanced

G

Gas exchange, Impaired
Grieving, Anticipatory
Grieving, Dysfunctional
Growth and development, Delayed
Growth, Risk for disproportionate

H

Health maintenance, Impaired
Health maintenance, Ineffective
Health-seeking behaviors
Hopelessness
Hyperthermia
Hypothermia

I

Identity, Disturbed personal
Incontinence, Functional urinary
Incontinence, Reflex urinary
Incontinence, Stress urinary
Incontinence, Total urinary
Incontinence, Urge urinary
Incontinence, Risk for urge urinary
Infant behavior, Disorganized
Infant behavior, Risk for disorganized
Infant behavior, Readiness for enhanced organized
Infant feeding pattern, Ineffective
Infection, Risk for
Injury, Risk for preoperative-positioning
Intracranial adaptive capacity, Decreased

K

Knowledge, Deficient

Knowledge, Readiness for enhanced

L

Lowliness, Risk for

M

Memory, Impaired

Mobility, Impaired bed

Mobility, Impaired physical

Mobility, Impaired wheelchair

N

Nausea

Neglect, Unilateral

Noncompliance

Nutrition: Less than body requirements, Imbalanced

Nutrition: More than body requirements, Imbalanced

Nutrition, Readiness for enhanced

Nutrition: More than body requirements, Risk for imbalanced

O

Oral mucous membrane, Impaired

P

Pain, Acute

Pain, Chronic

Parenting, Readiness for enhanced

Parenting, Impaired

Parenting, Risk for impaired

Peripheral neurovascular dysfunction, Risk for

Poisoning, Risk for

Post-trauma syndrome, Risk for

Powerlessness

Protection, Ineffective

R

Rape-trauma syndrome

Rape-trauma syndrome: Compound reaction

Rape-trauma syndrome: Silent reaction

Relocation stress syndrome

Relocation stress syndrome, Risk for

Role performance, Ineffective

S

Self-care deficit, Bathing/hygiene

Self-care deficit, Dressing/grooming

Self-care deficit, Feeding

Self-care deficit, Toileting

Self-concept, Readiness for enhanced

Self-esteem, Chronic law

Self-estccm, Situational law

Self-mutilation

Self-mutilation, Risk for

Sensory perception, Disturbed

Sexual dysfunction

Sexuality pattern, Ineffective

Skin integrity, Impaired

Sleep derivation

Sleep pattern, Disturbed

Sleep, Readiness for enhanced

Social interaction, Impaired

Social isolation

Sorrow, Chronic

Spiritual distress

Spiritual distress, Risk for

Spiritual well-being, Readiness for enhanced

Suffocation, Risk for

Suicide, Risk for

Surgical recovery, Delayed

Swallowing, Impaired

T

Therapeutic regimen management, Effective

Therapeutic regimen management, Ineffective

Therapeutic regimen management, Readiness for enhanced

Therapeutic regimen management, Ineffective community

Therapeutic regimen management, Ineffective family

Thermoregulation, Ineffective

Thought process, Disturbed

Tissue integrity, Impaired

Tissue perfusion, Ineffective

Transfer ability, Impaired

Trauma, Risk for

U

Urinary elimination, Impaired

Urinary alimentation, Readiness for enhanced

Urinary retention

V

Ventilation, Impaired spontaneous

Ventilator weaning response, Dysfunctional

Violence, Risk for other-directed

Violence, Risk for self-directed

W

Walking, Impaired

Wandering

Index